FIT FOR TWO

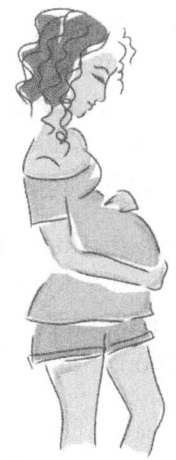

A Complete Exercise and Meal Plan Guide
for Expectant Mothers

Emily Coleman

TABLE OF CONTENTS

INTRODUCTION 7

Why Exercise and Nutrition are Important During Pregnancy

.... 10

Benefits of Exercise and Proper Nutrition for Both Mom and

Baby 13

    Benefits for Mom: 13

    Benefits for Baby: 14

    Integrating Workout and Good Nutrition into Pregnancy: 15

CHAPTER ONE 17

Body Changes and Nutrition During Pregnancy 17

    Changes in the Body During Pregnancy 19

    Nutrition Requirements During Pregnancy 21

    Macronutrients and Micronutrients for a Healthy Pregnancy

    23

CHAPTER TWO 27

Exercise During Pregnancy 27

    General Benefits of Exercise During Pregnancy 29

    Types of Exercise to Do and Avoid During Pregnancy 32

Sample Exercise Plan for Each Trimester 34

Tips for Safe and Effective Workouts 37

CHAPTER THREE 39

Meal Planning for a Healthy Pregnancy 39

Building a Balanced Pregnancy Meal Plan 41

Foods to Include and Avoid During Pregnancy 43

Meal Planning Tips for Each Trimester 46

Sample Meal Plans 49

Bonus: 30+ Days Meal Plan 52

CHAPTER FOUR 81

Managing Pregnancy Cravings and Aversions 81

Understanding Pregnancy Cravings and Aversions 82

Tips for Managing Cravings and Aversions 84

Healthy Alternatives for Common Cravings 86

CHAPTER FIVE 89

Special Considerations During Pregnancy 89

#Considerations for Women with Gestational Diabetes ... 92

#Considerations for Women with High Blood Pressure ... 94

#Considerations for Women with Multiples 96

#Considerations for Women with High-Risk Pregnancy.. 99

CHAPTER SIX 103

Postpartum Fitness and Nutrition.. 103

Advantages of Postpartum Fitness and Nutrition 104

Suggestions for Postpartum Exercise 105

Suggestions for Postpartum Nutrition............................. 106

Exercise Guidelines and Considerations After Pregnancy
.... 107

Nutrition Recommendations for Breastfeeding Moms ... 110

Sample Meal Plans for Postpartum Recovery 112

CONCLUSION 117

Maintaining a Healthy Lifestyle After Pregnancy 118

Final Thoughts and Encouragement 120

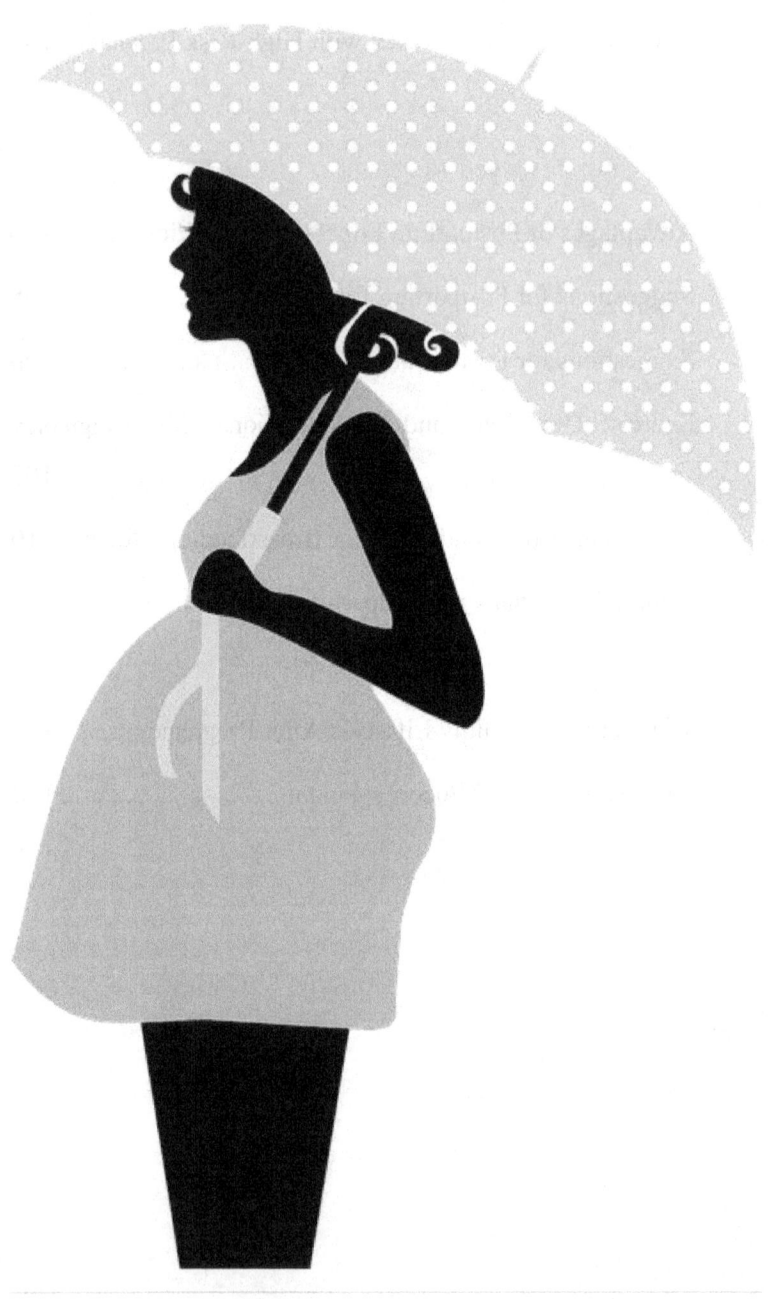

INTRODUCTION

"Fit for Two: A Complete Exercise and Meal Plan Guide for Expectant Mothers" is a complete handbook for pregnant moms who wish to be healthy and active throughout pregnancy. The book includes realistic advice on fitness and diet that is safe and helpful for both mom and baby. So how did the author come to compose this book? What encouraged her to assist other women to have a safe pregnancy?

Meet Emily, a first-time mom who learned the significance of fitness and diet throughout her pregnancy. Emily was happy when she found out she was pregnant, but also a bit scared. She understood that pregnancy would bring numerous changes to her body, but she didn't want to let that stop her from being active and healthy. She had always been an active person, and she wanted to continue to exercise and eat healthily for the sake of her developing kid.

At first, Emily found it tough to locate accurate information regarding fitness and diet during pregnancy. She wasn't sure what sorts of activities were safe, or how many calories she should be consuming each day. She sought online for direction but received contradicting suggestions that left her feeling confused and overwhelmed.

Eager to discover answers, Emily began reading books and scholarly articles regarding pregnancy and fitness. She spoke with her doctor and a trained dietician and slowly started to establish a strategy for keeping healthy and active throughout her pregnancy.

As she went through her pregnancy, Emily learned that exercise and diet not only helped her remain physically healthy but also emotionally strong. She discovered that exercise helped her manage stress and anxiety and that eating correctly provided her energy and enhanced her mood. She also saw that her infant looked to be prospering in her healthy surroundings.

Emily's pregnancy progressed successfully, and she gave birth to a healthy baby girl. But she didn't want to stop there. She wanted to share what she had learned with other pregnant women who may be struggling to find accurate information regarding fitness and diet during pregnancy. That's when she decided to publish Fit for Two: A Comprehensive Workout and Food Plan Guide for Expectant Moms.

In this book, Emily recounts her personal experiences and the research she did throughout her pregnancy. She gives practical advice and recommendations for exercising and eating healthily throughout each trimester, as well as specific concerns for women with high-risk pregnancies or gestational diabetes. She also gives examples of food plans and workout regimens that may be adapted to individual requirements and interests.

In her book, Emily seeks to educate pregnant moms to take ownership of their health and fitness throughout pregnancy. She wants women to know that they can have a healthy and active pregnancy and that doing so can benefit both mom and baby. She feels that by offering credible information and practical guidance, she may help other women experience the same excitement and confidence she felt throughout her pregnancy.

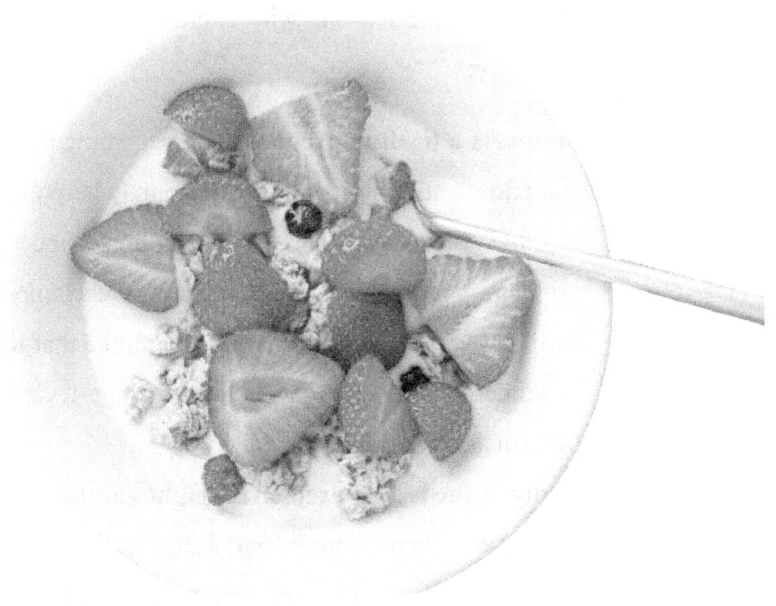

Importance of Exercise and Nutrition During Pregnancy

Pregnancy is a period of immense change and alteration for a woman's body. At this period, the body goes through several physiological and hormonal changes to support the growth and development of the baby. As such, pregnant moms must take additional care of their health and well-being throughout pregnancy, which includes keeping a balanced diet and indulging in regular exercise.

These are some of the reasons why exercise and diet are vital during pregnancy:

1. **Supports a healthy pregnancy:** Consuming a good diet and participating in regular exercise may help promote a healthy pregnancy. This may minimize the risk of problems such as gestational diabetes, preeclampsia, and early delivery. It may also assist guarantee that the baby is delivered at a healthy weight and with a lesser chance of birth abnormalities.

2. **Reduces the risk of excessive weight gain:** Pregnancy is a period when women naturally gain weight, but excessive weight gain may raise the risk of health issues for both the mother and baby. A good diet and regular

exercise may help women maintain a healthy weight throughout pregnancy and lower the risk of problems.

3. **Improves mood and decreases stress:** Exercise and a balanced diet may also have a favorable influence on mental health during pregnancy. It may help relieve tension and anxiety, boost mood, and encourage better sleep. This might be particularly essential for pregnant moms who may be experiencing mood swings or battling anxiety or sadness.

4. **Increases energy levels:** Pregnancy may be physically taxing, and many women suffer weariness at this time. A good diet and regular exercise may help raise energy levels and prevent weariness, making it simpler for pregnant women to perform their daily duties.

5. **Prepares the body for labor and delivery:** Regular exercise throughout pregnancy may also help prepare the body for labor and delivery. It helps enhance muscle tone and endurance, which can assist make the delivery procedure simpler and less traumatic for the body.

6. **Supports postpartum recovery:** A good diet and regular exercise may also assist promote a speedier and smoother postpartum recovery. It may help women restore their strength and energy after birth, and minimize the incidence of postpartum depression.

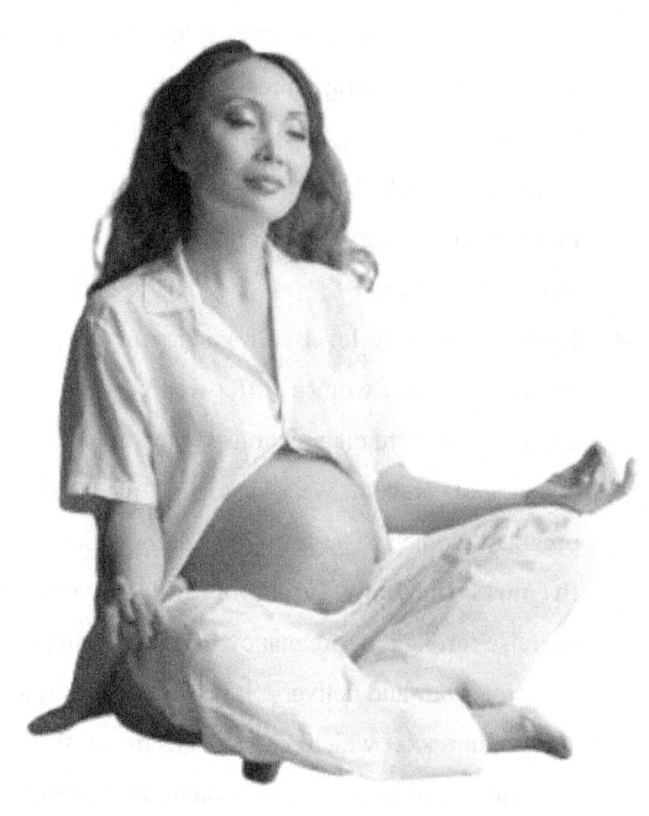

Benefits of Exercise and Proper Nutrition for Both Mom and Baby

Keeping a balanced diet and regular exercise regimen throughout pregnancy may offer several advantages for both pregnant moms and their newborns. These are some of the ways that exercise and a healthy diet may help both mom and baby during pregnancy:

Benefits for Mom:

1. **Decreased risk of gestational diabetes:** Gestational diabetes is a kind of diabetes that arises during pregnancy. It may raise the risk of issues for both mom and baby, including high blood pressure, premature labor, and birth abnormalities. Physical exercise and a nutritious diet may help lower the chance of developing gestational diabetes.

2. **Better cardiovascular health:** Pregnancy may put additional pressure on the heart and circulatory system. Participating in regular exercise may assist improve cardiovascular health and minimize the risk of issues such as high blood pressure and preeclampsia.

3. **Decreased risk of excessive weight gain:** Excessive weight gain during pregnancy may raise the risk of problems such as preterm delivery and gestational diabetes. A good diet and regular exercise may help avoid excessive weight gain and ensure a healthy pregnancy.

4. **Better mood and mental health:** Pregnancy may be a difficult and emotional period, and many women suffer mood swings or depression during this time. Exercise and an adequate diet may help enhance mood and decrease stress, encouraging improved mental health during pregnancy.

5. **Enhanced postpartum recovery:** Keeping a good diet and exercise regimen throughout pregnancy may aid improve postpartum recovery. It may help women restore their strength and stamina more rapidly after birth, and minimize the risk of postpartum depression.

Benefits for Baby:

1. **Reduced risk of birth defects:** A good diet and regular exercise throughout pregnancy may help lower the risk of birth problems such as spina bifida and heart defects.

2. **Reduced chance of preterm delivery:** Preterm birth is a serious worry for pregnant moms, since it may lead to

difficulties and long-term health concerns for the infant. Exercise and an appropriate diet may help minimize the risk of premature birth.

3. **Enhanced brain development:** A balanced diet during pregnancy may assist promote healthy brain development in the baby, supporting higher cognitive performance and minimizing the chance of developmental delays.

4. **Better birth weight:** Infants born to moms who maintain a good diet and exercise regimen throughout pregnancy are more likely to be delivered at a healthy weight, minimizing the risk of problems such as respiratory distress and hypoglycemia.

5. **Reduced risk of childhood obesity:** Children born to moms who maintain a good diet and exercise regimen throughout pregnancy are less likely to be fat later in life.

Integrating Workout and Good Nutrition into Pregnancy:

Pregnant moms must approach exercise and diet safely and healthily throughout pregnancy. Here are some recommendations for combining exercise and an appropriate diet during pregnancy:

1. **Speak to your doctor:** Before beginning any workout or diet regimen, it's crucial to chat with your doctor. They

can help you build a strategy that is safe and suitable for your unique requirements and health state.

2. **Strive for a balanced diet:** A healthy diet during pregnancy should contain a mix of fruits and vegetables, lean meats, whole grains, and healthy fats. It's also vital to avoid meals that are heavy in sugar, salt, or bad fats.

3. **Stay hydrated:** Drinking enough water is vital during pregnancy, as it may help avoid dehydration and improve good digestion.

4. **Select safe workouts:** Not all exercises are safe during pregnancy, so it's crucial to pick activities that are low-impact and low-risk. Swimming, walking, yoga, and strength training with low weights are all typically safe workouts for expecting moms.

5. **Listen to your body:** It's crucial to listen to your body throughout pregnancy and not push yourself too much. If you feel fatigued or uncomfortable during exercise, take a break or change the activity as required.

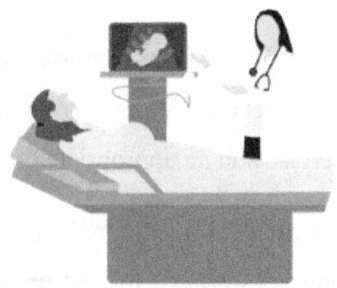

CHAPTER ONE

Body Changes and Nutrition During Pregnancy

Adequate nutrition throughout pregnancy is vital for both the mother and the growing child. It's crucial to maintain a well-balanced diet that contains a range of nutrients, such as protein, fiber, calcium, iron, and folic acid. These nutrients are crucial for proper fetal growth and may also help avoid issues during pregnancy, such as gestational diabetes and preeclampsia.

In addition to a balanced diet, frequent exercise may also be advantageous for expecting moms. Exercise may assist improve cardiovascular health, minimize the risk of excessive weight gain, and promote improved mental health during pregnancy. It may also help minimize the risk of problems such as gestational diabetes and premature childbirth.

Yet, it's crucial to approach exercise and diet safely and healthily throughout pregnancy. Some workouts may not be healthy during pregnancy, and it's crucial to contact a healthcare expert before beginning any new fitness plan. It's also vital to avoid some meals that may be detrimental to the growing baby, such as raw or undercooked meats, seafood rich in mercury, and unpasteurized dairy products.

Thankfully, there are numerous tools available to assist pregnant moms to navigate the realm of pregnancy fitness and nutrition. These options may include prenatal exercise programs, dietary advice, and internet resources like blogs and forums. Several healthcare practitioners also give counseling and assistance to pregnant women who are interested in maintaining a healthy lifestyle throughout pregnancy.

Ultimately, pregnant exercise and nutrition are about finding a balance that works for each particular expecting woman. By keeping educated, talking with healthcare specialists, and listening to their bodies, pregnant moms may stay healthy and active throughout pregnancy, and give their growing babies the nourishment and support they need for a successful start in life.

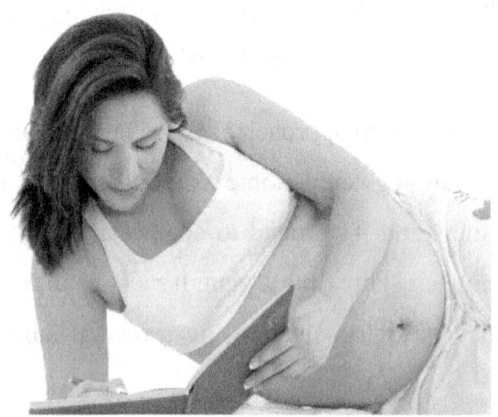

Changes in the Body During Pregnancy

Pregnancy is a unique and changing moment in a woman's life. As the body prepares for the growth and development of a new life, a range of changes occur that might impair a woman's physical and mental well-being. These are some of the significant changes that occur throughout pregnancy.

1. **Hormonal Changes:** Throughout pregnancy, a woman's body undergoes a spike in hormones such as estrogen and progesterone. These hormones play a critical role in preparing the body for pregnancy and delivery. They serve to thicken the lining of the uterus, control the menstrual cycle, and avoid premature contractions. Yet, these hormonal shifts may also contribute to a variety of symptoms such as nausea, exhaustion, and mood swings.

2. **Weight Gain:** While the baby grows and develops, a woman's body will naturally gain weight. This weight increase is vital for a healthy pregnancy, but it may also place significant pressure on the body. To promote a successful pregnancy, it's crucial for pregnant moms to monitor their weight increase and maintain a good diet and exercise regimen.

3. **Changes in the Reproductive System:** Throughout pregnancy, the reproductive system experiences a variety of modifications to support the growth and development

of the baby. The cervix and vaginal walls grow softer and more elastic, which might make sexual intercourse more pleasant. The uterus also swells to accommodate the developing baby, which may put pressure on the bladder and induce frequent urination.

4. **Changes in the Cardiovascular System:** While the body tries to support the growth and development of the baby, the cardiovascular system experiences a variety of changes. Blood volume rises, and the heart works harder to pump blood throughout the body. This may cause symptoms such as exhaustion, shortness of breath, and swelling in the hands and feet.

5. **Changes in the Digestive System:** During pregnancy, the digestive system slows down to allow for greater absorption of nutrients. This might lead to symptoms such as constipation, heartburn, and bloating. Moreover, the developing baby might exert pressure on the stomach and intestines, which can make it difficult to consume substantial meals.

6. **Changes in the Musculoskeletal System:** As the baby grows and develops, the body's musculoskeletal system likewise experiences modifications. The developing uterus may place strain on the pelvic bones and joints, which can contribute to discomfort and agony. Moreover,

the ligaments and joints in the body become more loosened in preparation for delivery, which might raise the risk of injury and strain.

In conclusion, pregnancy is a moment of deep change and transition in a woman's life. These changes are required for the growth and development of a healthy baby, but they may also impair a woman's physical and mental well-being. By keeping educated and working closely with their healthcare practitioner, pregnant moms may negotiate these changes and ensure a successful pregnancy and birthing.

Nutrition Requirements During Pregnancy

Good nutrition is vital for a healthy pregnancy and the growth and development of the baby. During pregnancy, a woman's body has increased dietary demands to maintain both her health and those of the developing baby. Following are some of the essential dietary needs during pregnancy:

1. **Protein:** Protein is important for the growth and development of the baby, as well as for the upkeep of the mother's tissues. During pregnancy, it's suggested that women take an extra 25 grams of protein each day. Excellent sources of protein include lean meats, poultry, fish, eggs, beans, and nuts.

2. **Folate:** Folate is a B vitamin that is necessary for the development of the neurological system in the baby. It's suggested that pregnant women get 600-800 mcg of folate each day, either via food or supplementation. Excellent sources of folate include leafy green vegetables, citrus fruits, legumes, and fortified cereals.

3. **Iron:** Iron is required to form hemoglobin, which transports oxygen in the blood. During pregnancy, iron demands rise to support the development of the baby and the expansion of the mother's blood volume. It's suggested that pregnant women ingest 27 mg of iron every day. Excellent sources of iron include red meat, chicken, fish, beans, and fortified grains.

4. **Calcium:** Calcium is needed for the development of strong bones and teeth in the baby, as well as for the preservation of the mother's bones. During pregnancy, it's suggested that women ingest 1000-1300 mg of calcium each day. Excellent sources of calcium include dairy products, leafy green vegetables, and fortified foods such as orange juice and tofu.

5. **Vitamin D:** Vitamin D is essential to help the body absorb calcium and support bone health. During pregnancy, it's suggested that women ingest 600-800 IU of vitamin D each day. Excellent sources of vitamin D

include fatty fish, egg yolks, and fortified foods such as milk and orange juice.

6. **Omega-3 Fatty Acids:** Omega-3 fatty acids are vital for the development of the embryonic brain and eyes. Throughout pregnancy, it's suggested that women ingest 200-300 mg of DHA (a form of omega-3 fatty acid) every day. Excellent sources of DHA include fatty fish, such as salmon and tuna.

In addition to these nutrients, it's crucial for pregnant women to keep hydrated and to eat a balanced diet that contains a range of fruits, vegetables, whole grains, and lean proteins. Pregnant women should also avoid alcohol, caffeine, and some kinds of seafood that are rich in mercury. Partnering with a healthcare physician or a qualified dietitian may give extra information and assistance for achieving dietary requirements throughout pregnancy.

Macronutrients and Micronutrients for a Healthy Pregnancy

Throughout pregnancy, both macronutrients and micronutrients play vital roles in sustaining the mother's health and fetal growth. Here's a summary of the important macronutrients and micronutrients required for a healthy pregnancy:

MACRONUTRIENTS:

1. **Carbohydrates:** Carbohydrates are a vital source of energy during pregnancy, and should make up roughly 45-65% of total daily calories. Healthy sources of carbs include whole grains, fruits, vegetables, and legumes.

2. **Protein:** Protein is vital for fetal growth and development, as well as for the preservation of maternal tissues. Pregnant women should take between 70-100 grams of protein per day, using sources such as lean meats, chicken, fish, eggs, dairy, and legumes.

3. **Fats:** Fats are vital for energy and the development of the embryonic brain and nervous system. Around 20-35% of total daily calories should come from healthy fats such as omega-3 fatty acids found in fish, nuts, seeds, and plant-based oils.

MICRONUTRIENTS:

1. **Folate:** Folate is a B vitamin that is important for fetal brain and nervous system development. Pregnant women should take at least 600-800 mcg of folate per day, which may be found in leafy greens, beans, fortified cereals, and supplements.

2. **Iron:** Iron is vital for fetal growth and development and for avoiding anemia in pregnant mothers. The daily recommended consumption for pregnant women is 27 milligrams per day, found in foods such as red meat, chicken, fish, beans, and fortified cereals.

3. **Calcium:** Calcium is vital for fetal bone growth and sustaining maternal bone health. Pregnant women should eat 1,000-1,300 mg of calcium per day, which may be found in dairy products, leafy greens, and fortified meals.

4. **Vitamin D:** Vitamin D is crucial for fetal bone growth and development, as well as maternal bone health. Pregnant women should ingest 600-800 IU of vitamin D per day, which may be found in fatty fish, egg yolks, and fortified foods.

5. **Zinc:** Zinc is crucial for fetal growth and development, as well as maternal immunological function. Pregnant women should ingest 11-13 mg of zinc per day, which may be found in meats, shellfish, whole grains, and nuts.

Pregnant women must have a balanced diet with a range of nutrient-dense foods to support their health and the growth and development of their babies. Engaging with a healthcare physician or certified dietitian may give extra information and assistance for fulfilling macronutrient and micronutrient demands throughout pregnancy.

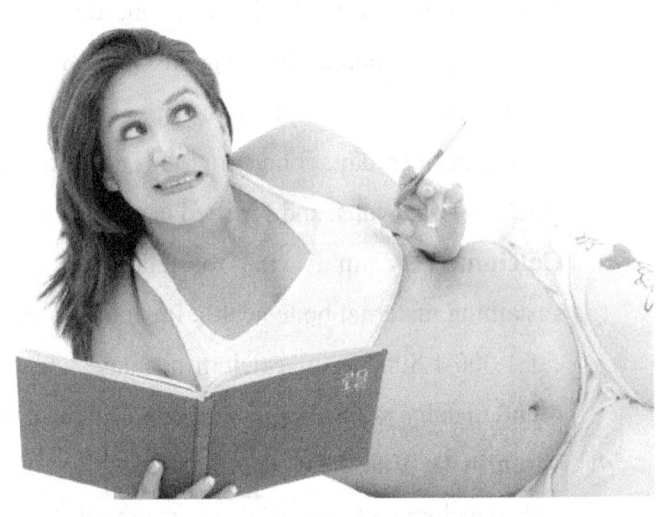

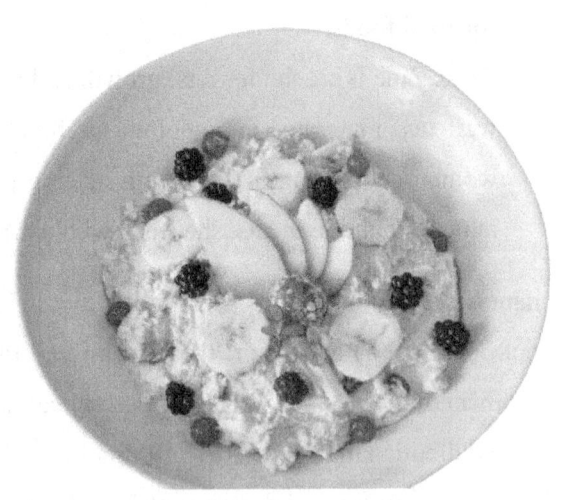

CHAPTER TWO

Exercise During Pregnancy

Exercise during pregnancy may offer various advantages for both the mother and the growing child, including better cardiovascular health, lower risk of gestational diabetes and preeclampsia, and improved mood and sleep. Nonetheless, it's crucial to exercise safely and correctly throughout pregnancy, since the body experiences major changes. These are some basic tips for exercising during pregnancy:

1. **Speak to your healthcare provider:** Before beginning or maintaining a fitness regimen during pregnancy, it's crucial to contact your healthcare professional to confirm that it's healthy for you and your growing baby.

2. **Select low-impact activities:** Activities like walking, swimming, cycling, and prenatal yoga are typically safe and useful during pregnancy. Avoid high-impact activities such as running or leaping, since these might place extra stress on the joints and pelvic floor.

3. **Listen to your body:** Throughout pregnancy, the body experiences major changes that might influence exercise tolerance. It's crucial to listen to your body and adapt your

workout program as required, such as taking pauses or lessening the intensity.

4. **Keep hydrated:** It's crucial to remain hydrated throughout the activity, particularly during pregnancy. Drink water before, during, and after exercise to help maintain hydration.

5. **Prevent overheating:** Overheating may be problematic during pregnancy since it can raise the chance of issues such as neural tube abnormalities. Avoid exercising in hot and humid surroundings, and wear loose, breathable clothes.

6. **Adjust as needed:** As the pregnancy continues, adaptations to the workout plan may be required to accommodate changes in the body. For example, utilizing a stability ball for balance during strength training, or adjusting yoga positions to suit an expanding belly.

7. **Pelvic floor exercises:** The pelvic floor muscles support the bladder, uterus, and colon, and may be compromised during pregnancy and delivery. Pelvic floor exercises, such as Kegels, may help strengthen these muscles and lower the risk of incontinence and other pelvic floor diseases.

Generally, exercise may be safe and useful during pregnancy, but it's crucial to speak with a healthcare expert and listen to your body. Strive for at least 150 minutes of moderate-intensity aerobic activity each week, and integrate strength training and stretching as well.

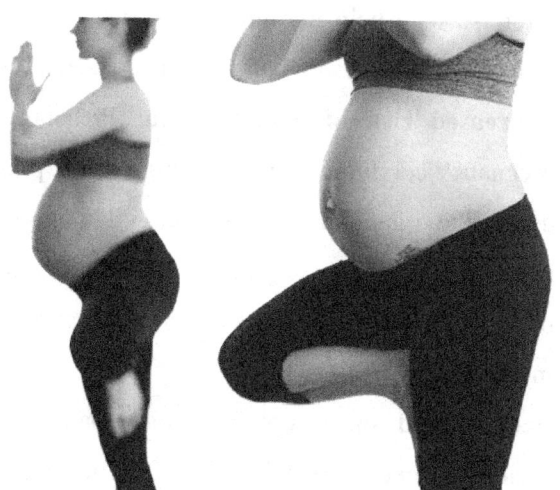

walking/ running 5X per wk

General Benefits of Exercise During Pregnancy

Exercising during pregnancy provides several advantages for both the mother and the growing child. These are some of the advantages of exercising during pregnancy:

1. **Increased cardiovascular health:** Exercise may help strengthen the heart and improve circulation, which is particularly essential during pregnancy when the body is working harder to give blood and nutrients to the growing baby.

2. **Decreased risk of gestational diabetes:** Gestational diabetes is a kind of diabetes that arises during pregnancy and may lead to difficulties for both the mother and baby. Exercise may help minimize the chance of developing gestational diabetes by boosting insulin sensitivity.

3. **Decreased risk of preeclampsia:** Preeclampsia is a pregnancy condition marked by high blood pressure and damage to organs such as the liver and kidneys. Exercise may help minimize the chance of developing preeclampsia by increasing circulation and decreasing inflammation.

4. **Better mood and sleep:** Pregnancy may be a difficult period, and exercise can help improve mood and decrease tension and anxiety. Exercise may also assist improve sleep quality, which is vital for general health and well-being during pregnancy.

5. **Decreased risk of excessive weight gain:** Excessive weight gain during pregnancy might raise the risk of issues such as gestational diabetes, preeclampsia, and delivery difficulties. Exercise may help lower the risk of excessive weight gain by boosting energy expenditure and supporting healthy eating habits.

6. **Increased strength and endurance:** Since the body experiences substantial changes during pregnancy,

including weight gain and changes in posture, exercise may assist enhance strength and endurance, which can help minimize the risk of musculoskeletal discomfort and improve overall function.

7. **Shorter labor and delivery:** Exercising throughout pregnancy may assist enhance the strength and endurance of the muscles used during labor and delivery, which can contribute to a shorter and simpler delivery.

Overall, exercise during pregnancy may have several advantages for both the mother and the growing child. It's crucial to check with a healthcare practitioner and follow safe exercise recommendations to maintain a healthy and safe pregnancy.

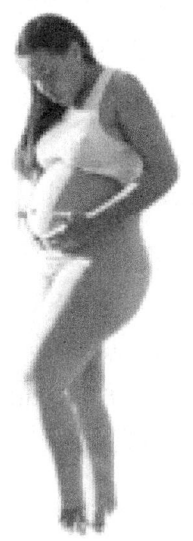

Types of Exercise to Do and Avoid During Pregnancy

Throughout pregnancy, it's crucial to pick workouts that are safe and suitable for the growing body. These are some sorts of workouts to consider, as well as those to avoid:

EXERCISES TO DO:

1. **Walking:** Walking is a low-impact activity that may be done throughout pregnancy. It's a terrific method to keep active and preserve cardiovascular health.

2. **Swimming:** Swimming is a fantastic low-impact workout that may assist improve cardiovascular health and general fitness. It's also a terrific method to remain cool and minimize edema during pregnancy.

3. **Pregnancy yoga:** Prenatal yoga may assist increase flexibility, strength, and balance. It may also help relieve stress and enhance general happiness.

4. **Strength training:** Strength training may help enhance muscular strength and endurance, which can help minimize the risk of musculoskeletal discomfort and improve overall function throughout pregnancy and postpartum.

5. **Pelvic floor exercises:** Pelvic floor exercises, such as Kegels, may help strengthen the pelvic floor muscles, which can lower the risk of incontinence and other pelvic floor diseases.

EXERCISES TO AVOID:

1. **High-impact activities:** High-impact workouts like jogging or leaping may place extra stress on the joints and pelvic floor, which can increase the risk of injury and difficulties during pregnancy.

2. **Contact sports:** Contact sports such as basketball or soccer should be avoided during pregnancy owing to the danger of falls or accidents.

3. **Activities that involve laying on the back:** Exercises that require lying on the back, such as crunches or sit-ups, should be avoided after the first trimester, since they may restrict blood supply to the growing baby.

4. **Hot yoga or hot pilates:** Hot yoga or hot pilates should be avoided during pregnancy, since overheating may be detrimental to the growing baby.

5. **Exercises that need holding the breath:** Activities that involve holding the breath, such as some forms of weightlifting, should be avoided during pregnancy, since they may elevate blood pressure and limit oxygen supply to the growing baby.

Generally, it's crucial to contact a healthcare physician before beginning or maintaining an exercise plan during pregnancy and to listen to your body and make modifications as required.

Sample Exercise Plan for Each Trimester

This is an example workout schedule for each trimester of pregnancy:

First Trimester:

Throughout the first trimester, it's crucial to concentrate on low-impact workouts and to listen to your body as it adapts to the changes of pregnancy.

Example workout plan:

- Walking: 20-30 minutes of brisk walking, 3-5 times a week.
- Prenatal yoga: 1-2 prenatal yoga courses each week.
- Pelvic floor exercises: 5-10 Kegel exercises, 2-3 times a day.

Second Trimester:

During the second trimester, it's crucial to continue with low-impact workouts, but you may also start introducing some strength training exercises to enhance muscular strength and endurance.

Example workout plan:

- Walking: 30-45 minutes of brisk walking, 3-5 times a week.
- Prenatal yoga: 1-2 prenatal yoga courses each week.
- Strength training: 2-3 days per week of resistance exercises, such as squats, lunges, and modified push-ups.
- Pelvic floor exercises: 10-15 Kegel exercises, 2-3 times a day.

Third Trimester:

Throughout the third trimester, it's vital to concentrate on workouts that are safe and pleasant, as the body prepares for labor and delivery.

Example workout plan:

- Walking: 20-30 minutes of brisk walking, 3-5 times a week.
- Prenatal yoga: 1-2 prenatal yoga courses each week.
- Strength training: 2 days per week of resistance exercises, such as squats, lunges, and modified push-ups.
- Pelvic floor exercises: 15-20 Kegel exercises, 2-3 times a day.

- Relaxation techniques: Employ relaxation methods, such as deep breathing or meditation, to decrease tension and increase relaxation.

It's crucial to listen to your body and make modifications to your fitness plan as required. Please speak with a healthcare physician before beginning or maintaining an exercise regimen during pregnancy.

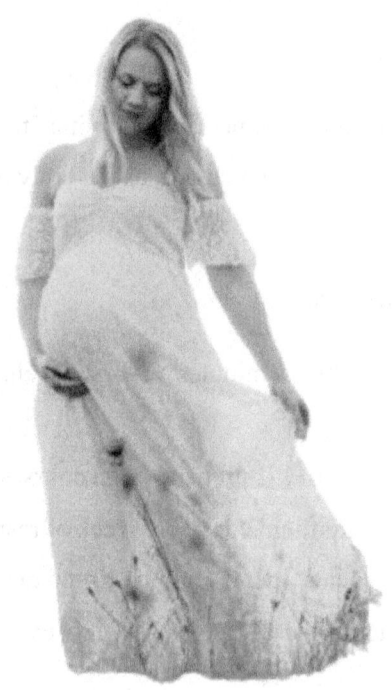

Tips for Safe and Effective Workouts

Here are some guidelines for safe and successful exercises during pregnancy:

1. **Talk with your healthcare provider:** Before beginning or continuing any fitness regimen during pregnancy, it's vital to speak with your healthcare provider to confirm that it's safe for you and your baby.

2. **Start slowly:** If you're new to fitness, start with low-impact activities, such as walking or swimming, and gradually increase the intensity and length of your exercises over time.

3. **Stay hydrated:** It's vital to drink enough water before, during, and after exercise to remain hydrated and avoid overheating.

4. **Choose comfortable clothes:** Select loose-fitting, comfortable clothing that allows for a full range of motion and gives support for your developing tummy.

5. **Employ appropriate form:** Proper form is vital for avoiding injury and getting the most out of your exercises. Try working with a trained pregnant exercise teacher who can educate you on the appropriate form and technique.

6. **Avoid high-risk activities:** Avoid activities that raise the risk of falls, such as contact sports or high-impact

activities, and avoid workouts that involve laying flat on your back after the first trimester.

7. **Listen to your body:** As your body changes throughout pregnancy, it's crucial to listen to your body and make modifications to your workout regimen as required. If you develop discomfort, dizziness, or shortness of breath, stop exercising and talk with your healthcare professional.

By following these suggestions, you may safely and efficiently include exercise into your pregnancy routine to maintain a healthy pregnancy and prepare your body for labor and delivery.

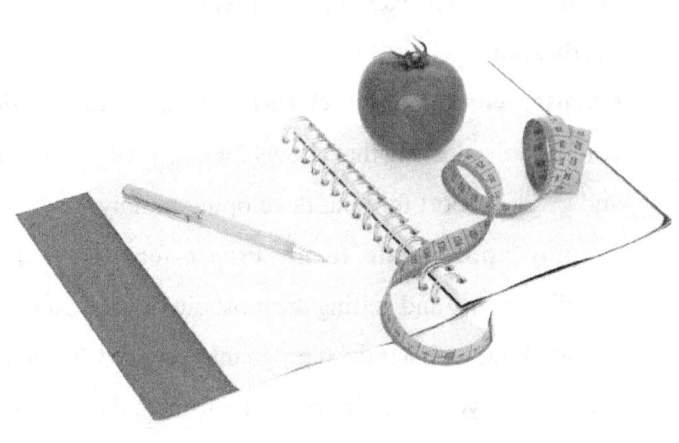

CHAPTER THREE

Meal Planning for a Healthy Pregnancy

Adequate nutrition during pregnancy is vital for the growth and development of the baby, as well as the health of the mother. Here are some recommendations for food planning for a healthy pregnancy:

1. **Concentrate on nutrient-dense foods:** Select foods that are high in nutrients, such as fruits, vegetables, whole grains, lean protein, and healthy fats.

2. **Consume a variety of meals:** Consuming a variety of foods guarantees that you're receiving a range of nutrients that are vital for a healthy pregnancy.

3. **Select foods high in folic acid:** Folic acid is vital for the development of the baby's neural tube. Select foods that are high in folic acids, such as leafy green vegetables, citrus fruits, and fortified grains.

4. **Incorporate sources of iron:** Iron is needed for the development of red blood cells, which supply oxygen to the baby. Select meals that are high in iron, such as lean red meat, chicken, fish, beans, and fortified cereals.

5. **Integrate sources of calcium:** Calcium is vital for the development of the baby's bones and teeth. Select foods that are high in calcium, such as dairy products, fortified plant milk, and leafy green vegetables.

6. **Minimize processed and high-sugar foods:** Processed and high-sugar diets may lead to excessive weight gain and raise the risk of gestational diabetes.

7. **Keep hydrated:** Drink lots of water throughout the day to remain hydrated and avoid constipation.

8. **Strive for small, regular meals:** Eating small, frequent meals throughout the day may help manage blood sugar levels and reduce nausea and heartburn.

By including these guidelines in your meal planning, you can guarantee that you're receiving the nutrients you need for a healthy pregnancy and a healthy baby. Consider working with a certified dietitian or healthcare practitioner to establish a tailored meal plan that suits your particular requirements and interests.

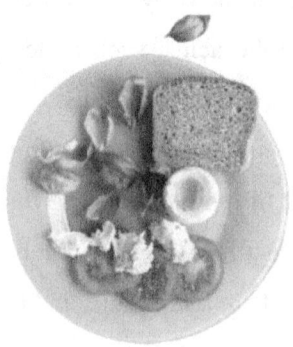

Building a Balanced Pregnancy Meal Plan

A balanced pregnancy meal plan should contain a range of nutrient-dense meals to ensure that both you and your baby are receiving the nutrients you need for a healthy pregnancy. Here's an example of a balanced pregnant food plan:

Breakfast:

- 1 cup of oats with sliced banana and chopped walnuts
- 1 cup of Greek yogurt
- 1 piece of whole-grain bread with peanut butter

Snack:

- 1 medium-sized apple
- 1 ounce of almonds

Lunch:

- Grilled chicken breast with roasted veggies (such as broccoli, carrots, and bell peppers)
- 1 cup of brown rice

1 cup of mixed greens with sliced cucumber and cherry tomatoes, seasoned with olive oil and balsamic vinegar

Snack:

- 1 cup of tiny carrots

- 2 teaspoons of hummus

Dinner:

- Baked salmon with steaming asparagus
- 1 medium-sized roasted sweet potato \s1 cup of mixed greens with sliced avocado, seasoned with lemon juice and olive oil

Snack:

- 1 cup of cut strawberries
- 1 ounce of dark chocolate

This meal plan offers a range of nutrient-dense foods, such as fruits, vegetables, whole grains, lean protein, and healthy fats. It also contains sources of critical nutrients for pregnancy, such as iron-rich lean protein, calcium-rich dairy products, and folic acid-rich leafy green vegetables.

Remember to drink lots of water throughout the day and to heed your body's hunger and fullness signals. Consider working with a certified dietitian or healthcare practitioner to establish a tailored meal plan that suits your particular requirements and interests.

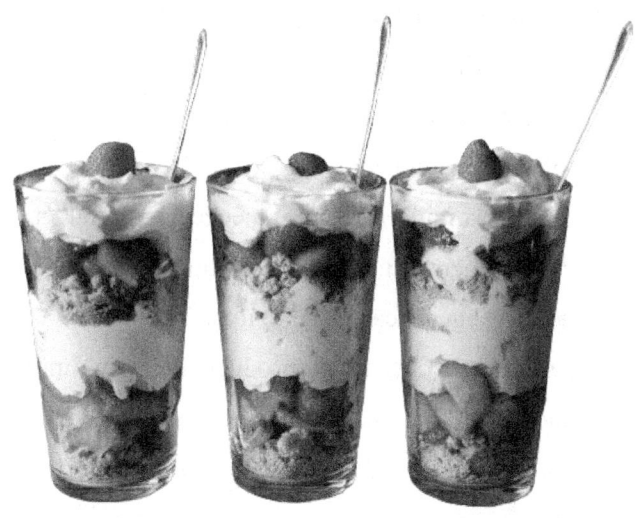

Foods to Include and Avoid During Pregnancy

Throughout pregnancy, it is crucial to pay great attention to the sorts of meals you ingest. Consuming a well-balanced diet is vital not just for your health but also for the growth of your kid. These are some items to eat and avoid during pregnancy:

FOODS TO INCLUDE:

1. **Fruits and Vegetables:** Fresh fruits and vegetables supply critical elements, including vitamins and minerals, that promote fetal growth and development. Strive for at least 5 servings of fruits and vegetables every day.

2. **Whole Grains:** Whole grains are an excellent source of fiber, which may help reduce constipation during pregnancy. Moreover, they include vital minerals such as folate, iron, and zinc.

3. **Lean Protein:** Protein is needed for fetal growth and development, and may be found in lean meats, fish, poultry, eggs, beans, and lentils.

4. **Low-Fat Dairy:** Dairy products including milk, yogurt, and cheese are wonderful sources of calcium, which is crucial for the development of your baby's bones and teeth.

5. **Healthy Fats:** Healthy fats such as those found in avocado, nuts, seeds, and olive oil are vital for brain development in the baby.

FOODS TO AVOID:

1. **High-Mercury Fish:** Some species, such as swordfish, shark, and king mackerel, have high amounts of mercury, which may be detrimental to the growing baby. Instead, choose low-mercury seafood such as salmon, shrimp, and canned light tuna.

2. **Raw or Undercooked Meat:** Eating raw or undercooked meat might put you at risk for foodborne infections such as listeria or toxoplasmosis, which can be detrimental to the developing baby.

3. **Unpasteurized Dairy:** Unpasteurized dairy products, such as soft cheeses like feta, brie, and blue cheese, might contain hazardous bacteria like listeria, which can cause miscarriage or stillbirth.

4. **Caffeine:** Although moderate doses of caffeine are typically safe during pregnancy, high caffeine consumption has been related to an increased risk of miscarriage and low birth weight. Try to restrict your caffeine consumption to 200mg or less per day.

5. **Alcohol:** There is no safe amount of alcohol intake during pregnancy. Consuming alcohol during pregnancy may raise the risk of fetal alcohol syndrome, which can cause physical and mental problems in the infant.

It is vital to speak with your healthcare physician about particular dietary guidelines during pregnancy. By maintaining a healthy and balanced diet, you can guarantee that you and your baby obtain the vital nutrients you need for a successful pregnancy.

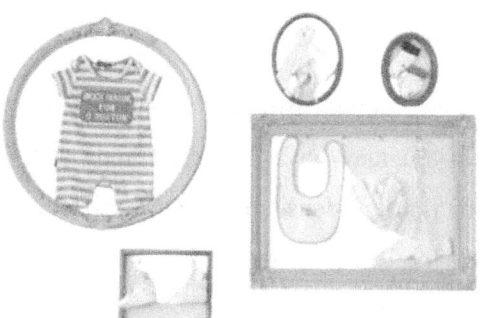

Meal Planning Tips for Each Trimester

Meal planning throughout pregnancy may be tough since your body and nutritional demands alter with each trimester. Here are some meal-planning recommendations for each trimester:

First Trimester:

During the first trimester, many women have morning sickness and may find it difficult to eat. It is crucial to concentrate on nutrient-dense diets and remain hydrated. Here are some tips:

Eat small, regular meals throughout the day instead of three big meals.

Select meals that are simple to digest, such as bland carbs (e.g., toast, crackers, rice).

Eat foods rich in vitamin B6, such as bananas, spinach, and chicken, since these may help ease nausea.

Second Trimester:

Throughout the second trimester, your energy levels may improve, and you may have increased hunger. It is crucial to concentrate on nutrient-dense diets that promote fetal growth and development. Here are some tips:

Strive for a balanced diet with a range of foods from all dietary categories.

Add sources of iron, such as lean red meat, dark leafy greens, and lentils, to support your increased blood volume.

Boost your diet with calcium-rich foods, such as dairy products, leafy greens, and fortified plant-based milk, to assist fetal bone and tooth development.

Third Trimester:

Throughout the third trimester, your baby is quickly developing and gaining weight. It is crucial to concentrate on nutrient-dense meals that promote your baby's growth and development. Here are some tips:

Boost your protein intake to assist fetal growth and development. Excellent sources of protein include lean meats, poultry, fish, eggs, and lentils.

Consume healthy fats, such as those found in nuts, seeds, avocados, and olive oil, to enhance embryonic brain development.

Concentrate on meals rich in fiber to avoid constipation and support good digestion. Excellent sources of fiber include fruits, vegetables, whole grains, and legumes.

In general, it is crucial to keep hydrated during all trimesters of pregnancy. Strive for at least 8 glasses of water every day and restrict your consumption of sugary beverages. Also, it is vital to avoid items that might be dangerous during pregnancy, such as raw or undercooked meats, unpasteurized dairy products, and high-mercury seafood.

Speak with your healthcare physician or a qualified dietitian for specific meal-planning assistance throughout pregnancy. By maintaining a balanced and nutrient-dense diet, you can promote a healthy pregnancy and the optimum growth of your kid.

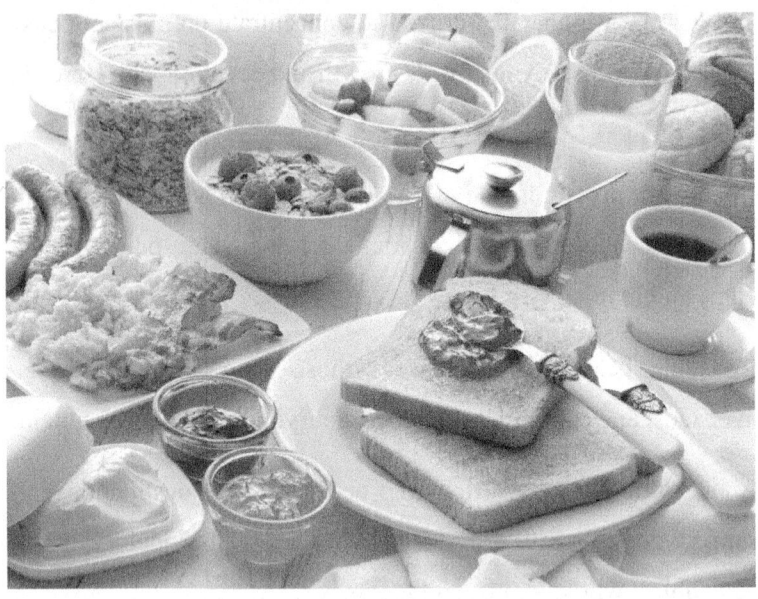

Sample Meal Plans

Here are three example meal plans for pregnant women:

Example Meal Plan 1

Breakfast:

- Greek yogurt with mixed berries and oats

Snack: Carrot sticks with hummus

Lunch:

- Grilled chicken salad with mixed greens, cherry tomatoes, avocado, and balsamic vinaigrette

Snack: Apple slices with almond butter

Dinner:

- Grilled salmon with quinoa and roasted veggies (such as bell peppers, zucchini, and onion)

Snack: Frozen grapes

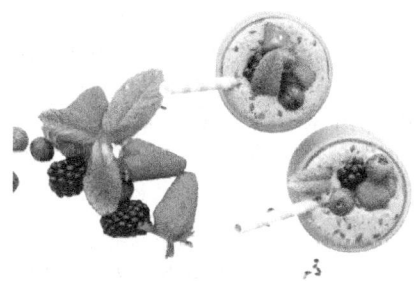

Example Meal Plan 2:

Breakfast:

- Whole grain bread with scrambled eggs and sliced avocado

Snack: Baby carrots with ranch dip

Lunch:

- Tuna salad on whole grain bread with lettuce and tomato

Snack: Trail mix with dried fruit and nuts

Dinner:

- Turkey chili with brown rice and a side salad

Snack: Greek yogurt with honey and chopped almonds

Example Meal Plan 3:

Breakfast:

- Oatmeal with banana slices and almond butter

Snack: Handmade trail mix with nuts, seeds, and dried fruit

Lunch:

- Vegetable stir-fry with tofu and brown rice

Snack: Orange slices with cottage cheese

Dinner:

- Grilled chicken kebabs with roasted sweet potatoes and broccoli

Snack: Dark chocolate-coated strawberries

Remember to contact your healthcare physician or a trained dietitian to design a tailored food plan that suits your requirements and preferences throughout pregnancy.

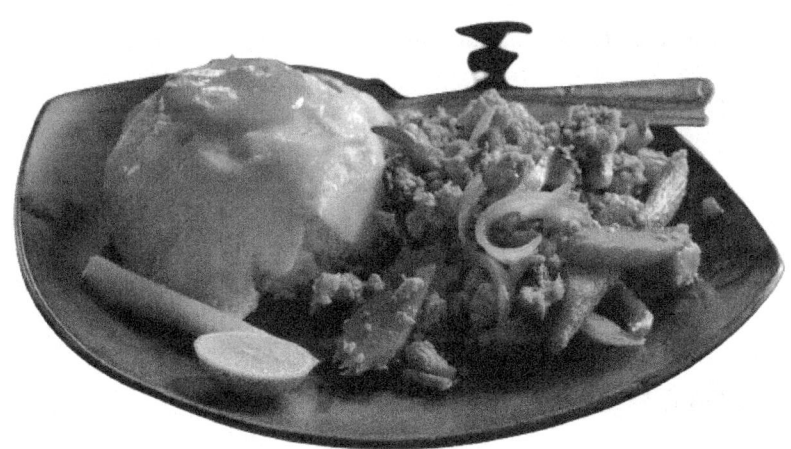

Bonus: 30+ Days Meal Plan

Here's a 30-day balanced pregnancy meal plan to help you get started with preparing healthy meals throughout your pregnancy:

DAY 1

Breakfast:

- Greek yogurt with mixed berries and granola

Snack: Apple slices with almond butter

Lunch:

- Grilled chicken with quinoa and roasted veggies

Snack: Carrots with hummus

Dinner:

- Baked salmon with sweet potato and green beans

Snack: Low-fat cottage cheese with pineapple chunks

DAY 2

Breakfast:

- Oatmeal with sliced banana and chopped walnuts

Snack: Orange slices with almonds

Lunch:

- Lentil soup with mixed greens and whole-grain bread

Snack: Edamame

Dinner:

- Turkey meatballs with zucchini noodles and tomato sauce

Snack: Low-fat plain yogurt with sliced kiwi

DAY 3

Breakfast:

- Scrambled eggs with spinach and whole-grain bread

Snack: Pear slices with cashews

Lunch:

- Tuna salad with mixed vegetables and whole-grain crackers

Snack: Baby carrots with ranch dressing

Dinner:

- Grilled steak with roasted Brussels sprouts and brown rice

Snack: Low-fat chocolate milk

DAY 4

Breakfast:

- Smoothie bowl with frozen mixed berries, Greek yogurt, and granola

Snack: Hard-boiled egg with celery sticks

Lunch:

- Vegetable stir-fry with tofu and brown rice

Snack: Cherry tomatoes with mozzarella cheese

Dinner:

- Roasted chicken with sweet potato fries and green salad

Snack: Low-fat cottage cheese with peach slices

DAY 5

Breakfast:

- Whole-grain waffles with mixed berries and low-fat whipped cream

Snack: Pineapple chunks with macadamia nuts

Lunch:

- Grilled shrimp with roasted veggies and quinoa

Snack: Cucumber slices with tzatziki sauce

Dinner:

- Baked salmon with roasted asparagus and brown rice

Snack: Low-fat plain yogurt with mixed fruit

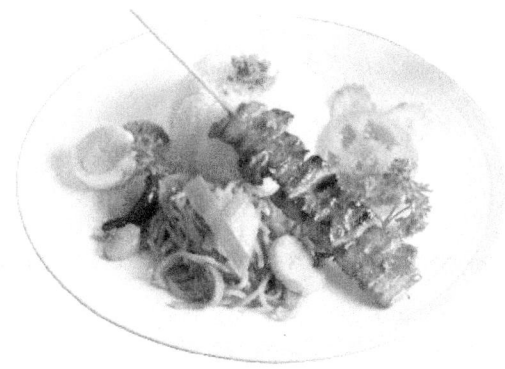

DAY 6

Brunch:

- Breakfast tortilla with scrambled eggs, black beans, and avocado

Snack: Banana slices with peanut butter

Lunch:

- Grilled chicken salad with mixed greens, cherry tomatoes, and balsamic vinaigrette

Snack: Trail mix with dried fruit and nuts

Dinner:

- Vegetable lasagne with a green salad

Snack: Low-fat chocolate pudding

DAY 7

Breakfast:

- Whole-grain pancakes with mixed berries and low-fat whipped cream

Snack: Mango slices with cashews

Lunch:

- Lentil and vegetable soup with whole-grain bread

Snack: Popcorn with grated Parmesan cheese

Dinner:

- Roasted chicken with roasted veggies and quinoa

Snack: Low-fat plain yogurt with mixed fruit

DAY 8

Breakfast:

- Greek yogurt with mixed berries and granola

Snack: Apple slices with almond butter

Lunch:

- Grilled salmon with roasted veggies and brown rice

Snack: Baby carrots with hummus

Dinner:

- Turkey chili with a green salad

Snack: Low-fat cottage cheese with pear slices

DAY 9

Breakfast:

- Oatmeal with sliced banana and chopped walnuts

Snack: Orange slices with almonds

Lunch:

- Grilled chicken with sweet potato and green beans

Snack: Edamame

Dinner:

- Baked tilapia with mixed vegetables and quinoa

Snack: Low-fat plain yogurt with mango chunks

DAY 10

Breakfast:

- Scrambled eggs with spinach and whole-grain bread

Snack: Grapefruit slices with cashews

Lunch:

- Vegetable soup with whole-grain bread

Snack: Cherry tomatoes with hummus

Dinner:

- Grilled steak with roasted Brussels sprouts and brown rice

Snack: Low-fat chocolate milk.

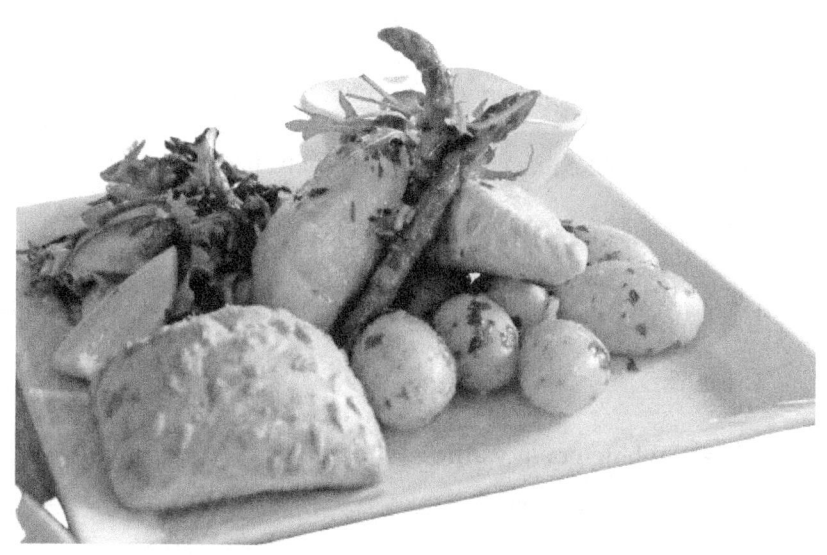

DAY 11

Breakfast:

- Smoothie bowl with frozen mixed berries, Greek yogurt, and granola

Snack: Hard-boiled egg with celery sticks

Lunch:

- Tuna salad with mixed vegetables and whole-grain crackers

Snack: Pineapple chunks with macadamia nuts

Dinner:

- Roasted chicken with sweet potato fries and green salad

Snack: Low-fat cottage cheese with peach slices

DAY 12

Breakfast:

- Whole-grain waffles with mixed berries and low-fat whipped cream

Snack: Banana slices with peanut butter

Lunch:

- Grilled shrimp with roasted veggies and quinoa

Snack: Cucumber slices with tzatziki sauce

Dinner:

- Vegetable stir-fry with tofu and brown rice

Snack: Low-fat plain yogurt with mixed fruit

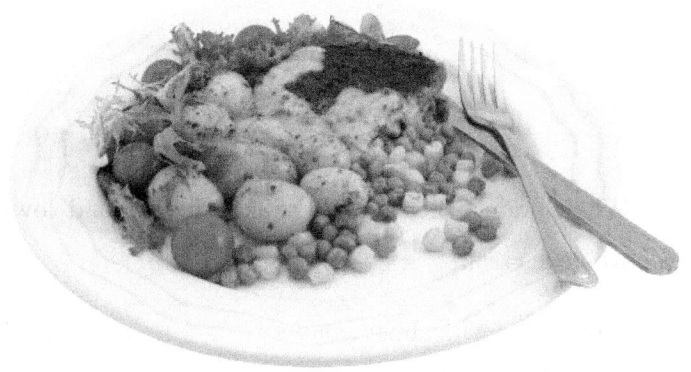

DAY 13

Brunch:

- Breakfast tortilla with scrambled eggs, black beans, and avocado

Snack: Mango slices with cashews

Lunch:

- Lentil and vegetable soup with whole-grain bread

Snack: Trail mix with dried fruit and nuts

Dinner:

- Baked salmon with roasted asparagus and brown rice

Snack: Low-fat chocolate pudding

DAY 14

Breakfast:

- Whole-grain pancakes with mixed berries and low-fat whipped cream

Snack: Apple slices with almond butter

Lunch:

- Grilled chicken salad with mixed greens, cherry tomatoes, and balsamic vinaigrette

Snack: Popcorn with grated Parmesan cheese

Dinner:

- Turkey meatballs with zucchini noodles and tomato sauce

Snack: Low-fat plain yogurt with mixed fruit

DAY 15

Breakfast:

- Greek yogurt with mixed berries and granola

Snack: Baby carrots with hummus

Lunch:

- Grilled salmon with roasted veggies and brown rice

Snack: Grapefruit slices with almonds

Dinner:

- Roasted chicken with sweet potato and green beans

Snack: Low-fat cottage cheese with mango chunks

DAY 16

Breakfast:

- Oatmeal with sliced banana and chopped walnuts

Snack: Orange slices with cashews

Lunch:

- Lentil soup with mixed greens and whole-grain bread

Snack: Edamame

Dinner:

- Baked tilapia with mixed vegetables and quinoa

Snack: Low-fat plain yogurt with pineapple chunks

DAY 17

Breakfast:

- Scrambled eggs with spinach and whole-grain bread

Snack: Pear slices with macadamia nuts

Lunch:

- Vegetable stir-fry with tofu and brown rice

Snack: Cherry tomatoes with hummus

Dinner:

- Grilled steak with roasted Brussels sprouts and brown rice

Snack: Low-fat chocolate milk

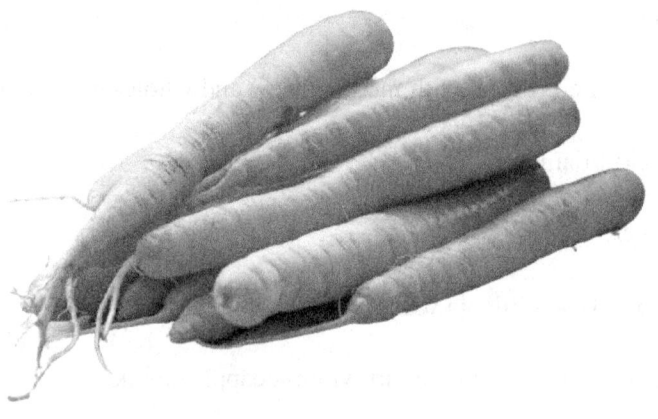

DAY 18

Breakfast:

- Smoothie bowl with frozen mixed berries, Greek yogurt, and granola

Snack: Hard-boiled egg with celery sticks

Lunch:

- Tuna salad with mixed vegetables and whole-grain crackers

Snack: Trail mix with dried fruit and nuts

Dinner:

- Roasted chicken with roasted veggies and quinoa

Snack: Low-fat cottage cheese with mixed fruit

DAY 19

Breakfast:

- Whole-grain waffles with mixed berries and low-fat whipped cream

Snack: Banana slices with almond butter

Lunch:

- Grilled shrimp with roasted veggies and quinoa

Snack: Cucumber slices with tzatziki sauce

Dinner:

- Vegetable lasagne with a green salad

Snack: Low-fat plain yogurt with kiwi slices

DAY 20

Breakfast:

- Greek yogurt with mixed berries and chopped almonds.
- Whole grain bread with mashed avocado and a fried egg

Lunch:

- Spinach and kale salad with grilled chicken, cherry tomatoes, sliced almonds, and balsamic vinaigrette.
- Whole grain crackers with hummus

Snack: Apple slices with almond butter. Hard-boiled egg

Dinner:

- Grilled salmon with quinoa and roasted Brussels sprouts

- Whole grain dinner roll

DAY 21

Breakfast:

- Oatmeal with mixed berries, chopped walnuts, and a drizzle of honey
- Green smoothie with spinach, banana, and almond milk

Lunch:

- Grilled chicken sandwich on whole grain bread with avocado, tomato, and lettuce
- Carrot sticks with hummus

Snack:

- Greek yogurt with sliced banana and granola
- Whole grain crackers with sliced cheese

Dinner:

- Grilled steak with roasted sweet potato and sautéed green beans
- Whole grain dinner roll

DAY 22

Breakfast:

- Scrambled eggs with spinach and whole grain toast
- Orange slices

Lunch:

- Quinoa salad with mixed veggies, chickpeas, and balsamic vinaigrette
- Apple slices with almond butter

Snack:

- Trail mix with mixed nuts and dry fruit
- Hard-boiled egg

Dinner:

- Roasted chicken with roasted carrots and mashed sweet potatoes
- Whole grain dinner roll

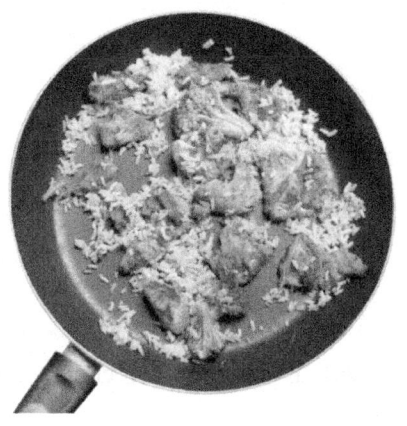

DAY 23

Breakfast:

- Greek yogurt with mixed berries and chopped walnuts
- Whole grain English muffin with mashed avocado and a fried egg

Lunch:

- Turkey and avocado wrap on whole grain tortilla with mixed vegetables and tomato
- Carrot sticks with hummus

Snack:

- Apple slices with almond butter
- Cheese stick

Dinner:

- Grilled prawns with brown rice and assorted veggies
- Whole grain dinner roll

DAY 24

Breakfast:

- Oatmeal with mixed berries, chopped walnuts, and a drizzle of honey
- Green smoothie with spinach, banana, and almond milk

Lunch:

- Spinach and kale salad with grilled chicken, cherry tomatoes, sliced almonds, and balsamic vinaigrette
- Whole grain crackers with hummus

Snack:

- Greek yogurt with sliced banana and granola
- Trail mix with mixed nuts and dry fruit

Dinner:

- Grilled chicken with quinoa and roasted Brussels sprouts
- Whole grain dinner roll

DAY 25

Breakfast:

- Scrambled eggs with spinach and whole grain toast
- Orange slices

Lunch:

- Quinoa salad with mixed veggies, chickpeas, and balsamic vinaigrette
- Hard-boiled egg

Snack:

- Carrot sticks with hummus
- Apple slices with almond butter

Dinner:

- Grilled steak with roasted sweet potato and sautéed green beans

Whole grain dinner roll

DAY 26

Breakfast:

- Greek yogurt with mixed berries and chopped almonds

- Whole grain English muffin with mashed avocado and a fried egg

Lunch:

- Grilled chicken sandwich on whole grain bread with avocado, tomato, and lettuce
- Whole grain crackers with hummus

Snack:

- Trail mix with mixed nuts and dry fruit
- Cheese stick

Dinner:

- Baked salmon with brown rice and mixed veggies
- Whole grain dinner roll

DAY 27

Breakfast:

- Greek yogurt with mixed berries, chia seeds, and honey.

Snack: Sliced cucumber and carrots with hummus.

Lunch:

- Whole wheat pita packed with grilled chicken, roasted veggies, and tzatziki sauce.

Snack: Apple slices with almond butter.

Dinner:

- Baked salmon with roasted asparagus and quinoa.

DAY 28

Breakfast:

- Scrambled eggs with spinach and whole wheat bread.

Snack: Greek yogurt with sliced peaches and granola.

Lunch:

- Spinach salad with grilled chicken, strawberries, feta cheese, and balsamic vinaigrette.

Snack: Raw almonds and an orange.

Dinner:

- Whole wheat spaghetti with turkey meatballs and tomato sauce.

DAY 29

Breakfast:

- Oatmeal with banana slices, walnuts, and cinnamon.

Snack: Sliced bell peppers with hummus.

Lunch:

- Whole wheat wraps with roasted turkey, avocado, spinach, and mustard.

Snack: Sliced apple with cheese.

Dinner:

- Grilled shrimp skewers with mixed veggies and brown rice.

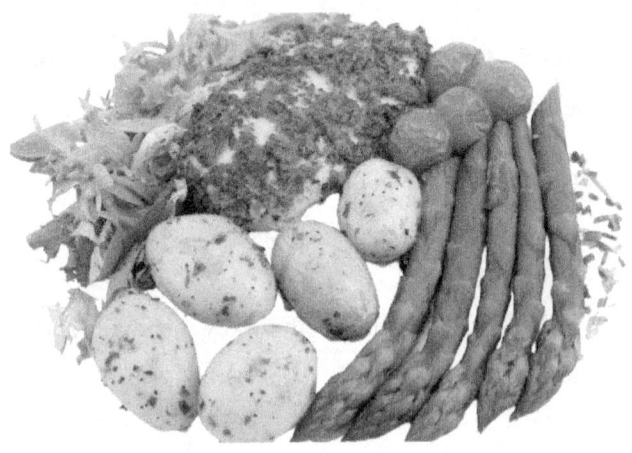

DAY 30

Breakfast:

- Greek yogurt with mixed berries, sliced almonds, and honey.

Snack: Raw carrots with tzatziki sauce.

Lunch:

- Roasted sweet potato with black beans, salsa, and plain Greek yogurt.

Snack: Orange slices and a hard-boiled egg.

Dinner:

- Baked chicken breast with roasted broccoli and brown rice.

DAY 31

Breakfast:

- Whole wheat English muffin with scrambled eggs, spinach, and tomato.

Snack: Sliced cucumber with hummus.

Lunch:

- Grilled chicken salad with mixed greens, cherry tomatoes, avocado, and balsamic vinaigrette.

Snack: Greek yogurt with mixed berries and granola.

Dinner:

- Baked cod with roasted Brussels sprouts and quinoa.

DAY 32

Breakfast:

- Smoothie with mixed berries, banana, Greek yogurt, and almond milk.

Snack: Raw almonds and an apple.

Lunch: Whole wheat pita loaded with tuna salad, lettuce, and tomato.

Snack: Sliced bell peppers with hummus.

Dinner:

- Grilled chicken kebabs with mixed veggies and brown rice.

DAY 33

Breakfast:

- Whole wheat bread with avocado and sliced hard-boiled egg.

Snack: Greek yogurt with sliced peaches and granola.

Lunch:

- Spinach salad with grilled chicken, strawberries, feta cheese, and balsamic vinaigrette.

Snack: Sliced cucumber with tzatziki sauce.

Dinner:

- Baked salmon with roasted asparagus and quinoa.

DAY 34

Breakfast:

- Oatmeal with banana slices, walnuts, and cinnamon.

Snack: Raw carrots with hummus.

Lunch:

- Whole wheat wraps with roasted turkey, avocado, spinach, and mustard.

Snack: Sliced apple with cheese.

Dinner:

- Whole wheat spaghetti with turkey meatballs and tomato sauce.

DAY 35

Breakfast:

- Greek yogurt with mixed berries, sliced almonds, and honey.

Snack: Sliced bell peppers with hummus.

Lunch:

- Grilled chicken salad with mixed greens, cherry tomatoes, avocado, and balsamic vinaigrette.

Snack: Orange slices and a hard-boiled egg.

Dinner:

- Baked chicken breast with roasted broccoli and brown rice.

DAY 36

Breakfast:

- Smoothie with mixed berries, banana, Greek yogurt, and almond milk.

Snack: Raw almonds and an apple.

Lunch:

- Roasted sweet potato with black beans, salsa, and plain Greek yogurt.

Snack: Greek yogurt with mixed berries and granola.

Dinner:

- Grilled shrimp skewers with mixed veggies and brown rice.

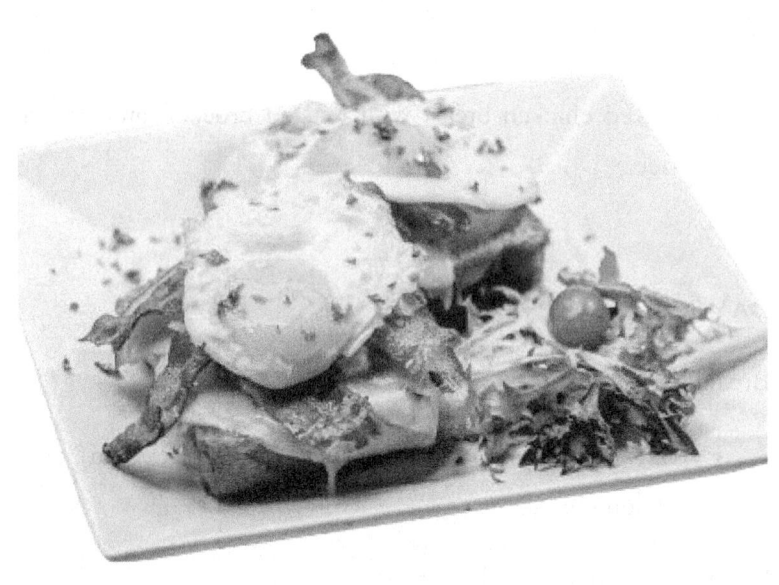

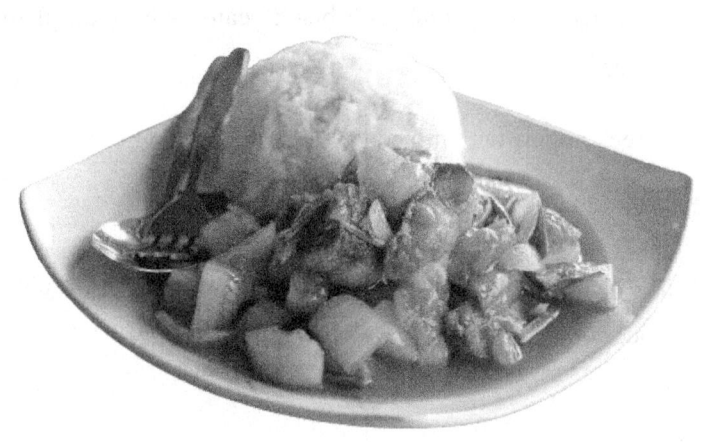

CHAPTER FOUR

Managing Pregnancy Cravings and Aversions

Pregnancy may be a period of significant dietary desires and aversions. Some women may suddenly seek things they never liked before, while others may find themselves unable to consume items they previously like. Handling these changes in appetite may be tough, but there are techniques to help you eat properly throughout pregnancy.

Initially, it is necessary to understand the causes underlying these desires and aversions. Hormone changes in pregnancy may create swings in appetite and affect your perception of taste and smell. Also, your body may be indicating that it requires particular nutrients, leading to specific food desires.

Although it is normal to indulge in odd yearning, it is crucial to maintain a balanced and healthy diet during pregnancy. This includes emphasizing nutrient-dense foods like fruits, vegetables, whole grains, lean meats, and healthy fats. These foods supply the vitamins, minerals, and macronutrients essential for a healthy pregnancy.

Understanding Pregnancy Cravings and Aversions

Prenatal cravings and aversions are normal and may be a cause of stress and bewilderment for many pregnant moms. These fluctuations in appetite may be caused by some variables, including hormonal shifts, dietary inadequacies, and psychological concerns.

Pregnancy cravings are often acute urges for certain foods or tastes. These desires might be for sweet, salty, sour, or spicy foods and can vary from moderate to powerful. Although the specific source of pregnant cravings is not understood, it is assumed that hormone changes have a role. For example, the hormone progesterone may change taste and scent, making some meals more tempting or unappetizing.

Prenatal aversions, on the other hand, are intense emotions of disgust or nausea towards particular foods or scents. These aversions might be to meals that were previously appreciated or to new foods. Like urges, the specific reason for pregnancy aversions is not understood but is thought to be connected to hormonal changes and a heightened sense of smell.

Although pregnant cravings and aversions are common, it is vital to be conscious of your nutrition and ensure that you are receiving the nutrients you and your baby need. If your desires are for harmful meals, attempt to discover healthier alternatives or enjoy them in moderation. If you are having aversions to nutrient-dense meals, consider introducing comparable but different foods into your diet or talk to a healthcare physician or qualified dietitian for help.

It is also crucial to realize that not all appetites and aversions are connected to food. Some women may develop cravings or aversions to non-food objects, such as dirt or chalk. This disorder, known as pica, may be hazardous and should be examined by a healthcare expert.

Overall, recognizing pregnancy cravings and aversions is vital for keeping a healthy and balanced diet throughout pregnancy. By being conscious of your nutrition and seeking counsel when required, you can help guarantee the health and well-being of you and your developing baby.

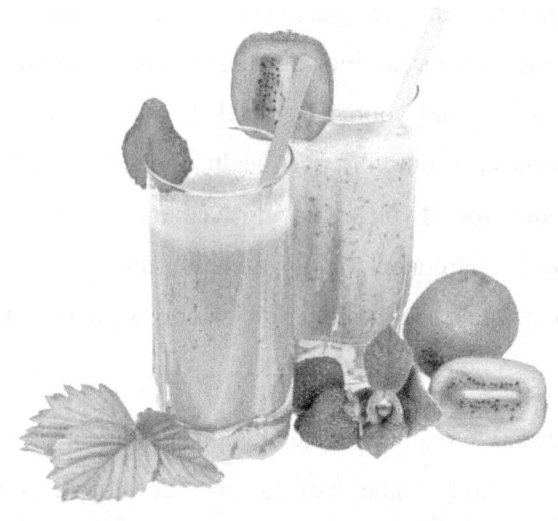

Tips for Managing Cravings and Aversions

Here are some strategies for controlling pregnant cravings and aversions:

1. **Have nutritious snacks on hand:** It is vital to be prepared for cravings by having healthy snack alternatives handy. Try to pick nutrient-dense snacks like fruits, veggies, nuts, and whole-grain crackers.

2. **Exercise moderation:** Although it is appropriate to indulge in urges from time to time, strive to practice moderation. For example, if you are seeking something

sweet, try a tiny piece of dark chocolate instead of a whole candy bar.

3. **Try with tastes:** If you are suffering from food aversions, attempt to experiment with various flavors and cooking techniques. For example, if you are opposed to raw veggies, consider roasting them instead.

4. **Keep hydrated:** Sometimes desires might be a consequence of dehydration. Make sure you are keeping hydrated throughout the day by drinking lots of water and other drinks.

5. **Seek alternatives:** If you are seeking something unhealthy, attempt to locate a healthier option. For example, if you are wanting ice cream, consider eating a small serving of Greek yogurt topped with fruit instead.

6. **Talk to your healthcare provider:** If you are having extreme or unusual cravings or aversions, speak to your healthcare provider. They may be able to give extra advice and help.

7. **Employ self-care:** Pregnancy may be a difficult time, and stress can intensify desires and aversions. Be sure to exercise self-care by getting adequate rest, keeping active, and doing things that help you relax and destress.

Remember, desires and aversions are typical aspects of pregnancy. By being attentive to your nutrition and getting help when required, you can manage these changes and maintain a healthy and balanced diet throughout your pregnancy.

Healthy Alternatives for Common Cravings

Pregnancy cravings may be a problem, particularly when you're attempting to maintain a healthy and balanced diet. Thankfully, many healthy alternatives to typical pregnancy cravings may help satisfy your sweet tooth or savory desires without jeopardizing your health or the well-being of your baby.

Here are some healthy alternatives to typical pregnancy cravings:

1. **Ice cream:** Instead of indulging in full-fat ice cream, consider enjoying a small dish of Greek yogurt topped with fresh fruit or a tiny handful of frozen grapes. Frozen yogurt or low-fat sorbet might also be suitable choices.

2. **Chocolate:** Dark chocolate may be a healthier alternative to milk chocolate or other sweet pleasures. Seek high-quality dark chocolate that includes at least 70% cacao for maximum health benefits. You may also try creating your own chocolate-dipped fruit or protein balls.

3. **Potato chips:** Instead of fried potato chips, try baked sweet potato chips or kale chips. These products are lower in fat and calories and provide more nutrients than typical potato chips.

4. **Candy:** Instead of grabbing for sweet candy, consider eating a piece of fruit, such as an apple or a banana, or a small portion of dry fruit like dates or raisins. These solutions are natural sources of sweetness and give more nutrients than sweets.

5. **Soda:** Instead of sugary soda, try sparkling water with a dash of fruit juice or slices of fresh fruit. You may also try creating your iced tea or flavored water with fresh herbs and fruit.

6. **Pizza:** Instead of buying fatty takeaway pizza, consider creating your pizza with a whole-wheat crust and lots of vegetables. You may also experiment with other toppings, such as grilled chicken or shrimp, to provide extra protein to your lunch.

7. **Burgers:** Instead of fast-food burgers, consider cooking your lean protein, such as turkey or chicken breast, and putting it on a whole-grain bun with lots of vegetables. You may also experiment with various condiments, like avocado or hummus, to add taste and nutrients to your meal.

Remember, pregnancy cravings are common and it's alright to indulge from time to time. Nonetheless, it's crucial to emphasize nutrient-dense diets and avoid extra sugar, salt, and saturated fat. By making smart choices and discovering alternatives to your favorite sweets, you may maintain a healthy and balanced diet throughout your pregnancy.

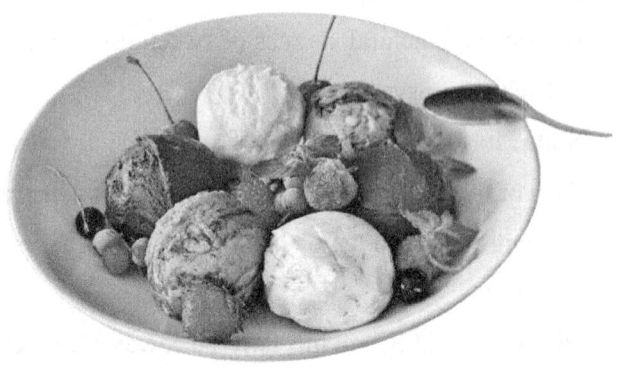

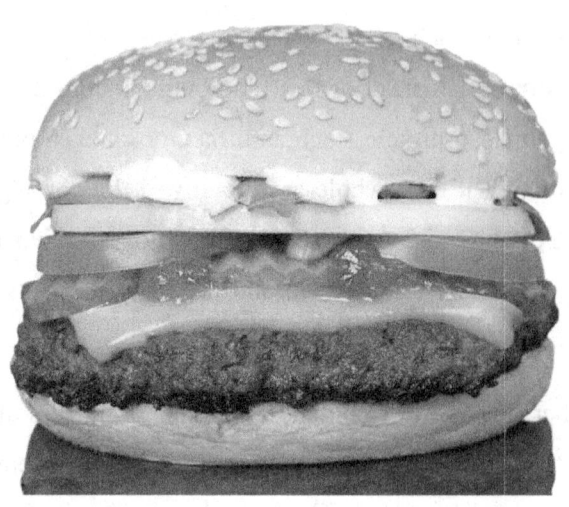

CHAPTER FIVE

Special Considerations During Pregnancy

Pregnancy is a period of substantial change in a woman's body, and there are unique concerns that should be taken into account to ensure a good pregnancy. These are some of the most significant points to bear in mind:

1. **High-risk pregnancies:** Certain pregnancies are deemed high-risk owing to pre-existing medical issues, age, or other circumstances. High-risk pregnancies need careful monitoring and may require extra care from a specialist.

2. **Prenatal care:** Proper prenatal care is vital to protect the health of both the mother and baby. Prenatal care comprises frequent appointments with a healthcare practitioner, ultrasounds, and numerous tests to monitor the health of the mother and baby.

3. **Medications:** Some drugs may be detrimental to the growing baby and should be avoided during pregnancy. It's crucial to consult a healthcare practitioner before taking any drugs, including over-the-counter pharmaceuticals and herbal supplements.

4. **Smoking, alcohol, and drugs:** Smoking, drinking alcohol, and taking drugs during pregnancy may have substantial detrimental impacts on the health of the growing baby. Some drugs should be avoided during pregnancy.

5. **Activity:** Exercise is typically safe and useful during pregnancy, but it's crucial to follow rules for safe exercise during pregnancy. High-impact workouts and exercises that entail reclining on the back should be avoided after the first trimester.

6. **Relax:** Rest is also crucial throughout pregnancy, particularly during the latter stages when the body is working hard to maintain the developing baby. Women should strive for 7-9 hours of sleep each night and take pauses during the day to relax.

7. **Nutrition:** Adequate nutrition is vital for the health of the growing baby and the mother. Pregnant women should strive for a balanced diet that contains lots of fruits, vegetables, whole grains, lean protein, and healthy fats. Some meals, such as raw or undercooked meat and fish, should be avoided during pregnancy.

8. **Mental health:** Pregnancy may be an emotional period, and it's crucial to consider mental health. Pregnant women

should seek help from family, friends, or a mental health professional if required.

In summary, there are numerous unique concerns to bear in mind throughout pregnancy to ensure a successful pregnancy and delivery. Women should work together with their healthcare practitioners to design a plan that suits their particular requirements and improves the health of both the mother and baby.

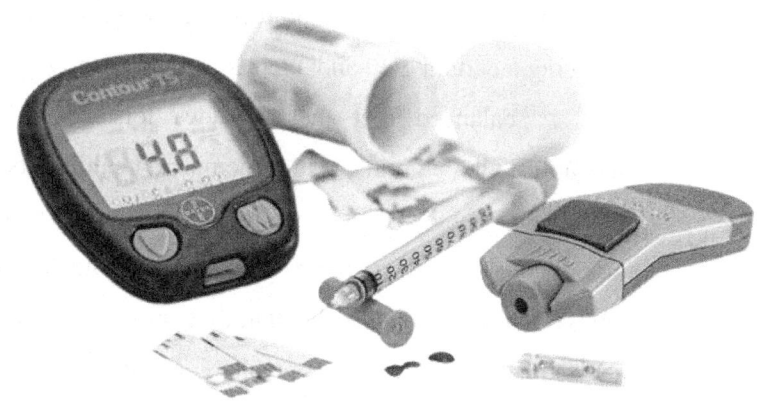

#Exercise and Nutrition Considerations for Women with Gestational Diabetes

Gestational diabetes is a kind of diabetes that arises during pregnancy. It may impair the health of both the mother and baby, but with good treatment, most women with gestational diabetes can have a successful pregnancy and birth. Activity and diet have a key role in the control of gestational diabetes. These are some concerns for women with gestational diabetes:

1. **Talk with a healthcare professional:** Women with gestational diabetes should work closely with a healthcare practitioner to build a strategy for managing their condition. This may entail monitoring blood sugar levels, following a certain diet, and exercising consistently.

2. **Diet:** A balanced diet that includes lots of fruits, vegetables, whole grains, lean protein, and healthy fats is crucial for women with gestational diabetes. Women should consult with a trained dietitian or a healthcare professional to design a food plan that suits their unique requirements and encourages stable blood sugar levels.

3. **Scheduling of meals and snacks:** Eating regularly spaced meals and snacks may help reduce blood sugar spikes and drops. Women with gestational diabetes should attempt to consume three meals and three snacks per day, with snacks spaced between meals.

4. **Activity:** Exercise may assist improve blood sugar management and general health during pregnancy. Women with gestational diabetes should attempt to exercise for at least 30 minutes each day, most days of the week. Low-impact workouts including walking, swimming, and yoga are often safe and useful for women with gestational diabetes.

5. **Monitoring blood sugar levels:** Women with gestational diabetes may need to check their blood sugar levels at home using a blood glucose meter. This may help them monitor their progress and make modifications to their diet and exercise program as required.

6. **Medications:** In certain situations, women with gestational diabetes may need to take medication to assist regulate their blood sugar levels. This should be done under the advice of a healthcare practitioner.

In short, women with gestational diabetes should engage closely with a healthcare physician to build a strategy for treating their disease. This may entail following a certain diet, exercising frequently, checking blood sugar levels, and taking medication as required. With adequate treatment, most women with gestational diabetes may have a successful pregnancy and delivery.

#Exercise and Nutrition Considerations for Women with High Blood Pressure

High blood pressure, or hypertension, is a common health problem that affects many women during pregnancy. It is vital for women with high blood pressure to maintain their condition with regular exercise and diet to avoid difficulties during pregnancy. These are some concerns for ladies with high blood pressure:

1. **Talk with a healthcare professional:** Women with high blood pressure should work closely with a healthcare practitioner to build a strategy for managing their condition. This may entail monitoring blood pressure levels, maintaining a certain diet, and exercising frequently.

2. **Diet:** A nutritious, well-balanced diet that is low in sodium and rich in potassium may help control high blood pressure during pregnancy. Women should engage with a trained dietitian or a healthcare professional to design a meal plan that suits their unique requirements and encourages stable blood pressure levels.

3. **Exercise:** Regular exercise may assist improve blood pressure management and general health during pregnancy. Women with high blood pressure should

strive to exercise for at least 30 minutes each day, most days of the week. Low-impact workouts such as walking, swimming, and yoga are often safe and useful for women with high blood pressure.

4. **Monitoring blood pressure levels:** Women with high blood pressure may need to check their blood pressure levels at home with a blood pressure monitor. This may help them monitor their progress and make modifications to their diet and exercise program as required.

5. **Medications:** In certain circumstances, women with high blood pressure may need to take medication to assist regulate their blood pressure levels. This should be done under the advice of a healthcare practitioner.

6. **Avoid specific foods:** Women with high blood pressure should avoid items that are rich in sodium, such as processed meals, fast food, and canned products. They should also avoid coffee since it might elevate blood pressure.

In summary, women with high blood pressure should work closely with a healthcare professional to build a strategy for managing their condition throughout pregnancy. This may involve following a certain diet, exercising frequently, monitoring blood pressure levels, and taking medication as required. By treating their high blood pressure, women may have a successful pregnancy and delivery.

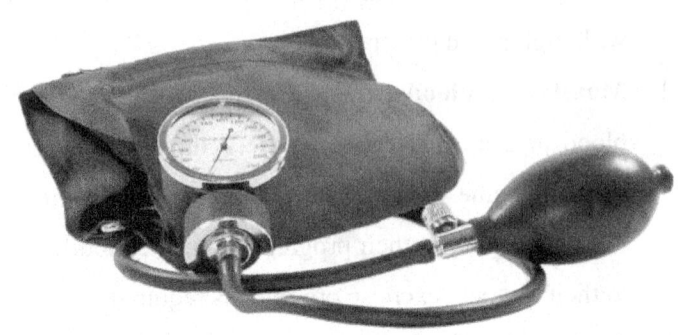

#Exercise and Nutrition Considerations for Women with Multiples

Pregnancy with multiples, such as twins or triplets, may provide particular obstacles when it comes to fitness and diet. These are some concerns for women bearing multiples:

1. **Talk with a healthcare professional:** Women carrying multiples should work closely with a healthcare practitioner to build a strategy for managing their pregnancy. This may entail monitoring weight growth, maintaining a certain diet, and exercising consistently.

2. **Diet:** A healthy, well-balanced diet is vital for women carrying multiple. Women should attempt to consume a

range of meals from all food categories to ensure they are receiving the nutrients they need for a healthy pregnancy. Women having multiples may need to eat more calories than women carrying a single kid, although the quantity may vary based on their specific circumstances. A licensed dietician can assist establish a food plan that matches their requirements.

3. **Exercise:** Frequent exercise may assist improve general health throughout pregnancy, although women carrying multiples may need to adapt their exercise program as their pregnancy advances. Low-impact workouts including walking, swimming, and prenatal yoga may be suitable, but high-impact exercises should be avoided. Women carrying multiples should check with their healthcare physician before commencing an exercise regimen.

4. **Monitoring weight increase:** Women having multiples may need to check their weight growth more carefully than women carrying a single kid. Women should strive to gain weight at a regular rate during their pregnancy, although the quantity of weight increase will vary based on their specific circumstances. Healthcare practitioners may assist select an acceptable weight gain target.

5. **Rest:** Women having multiples may require more rest than women carrying a single kid. It is crucial to listen to the body and relax when required to avoid difficulties during pregnancy.

6. **Preterm labor:** Women carrying multiples are at increased risk for preterm labor and should be aware of the signs and symptoms. They should talk with their healthcare physician and prepare a strategy for treating preterm labor if it arises.

In short, women carrying multiples should work closely with a healthcare physician to build a strategy for managing their pregnancy. This may involve following a particular diet, changing their exercise regimen, monitoring weight growth, relaxing when required, and preparing for premature labor. By taking these concerns into account, women bearing multiples may have a successful pregnancy and birth.

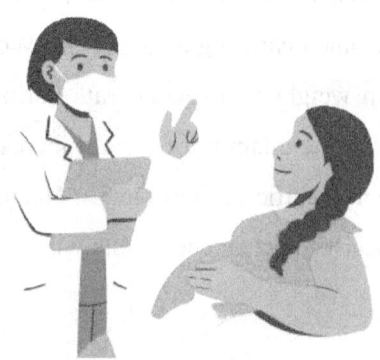

#Exercise and Nutrition Considerations for Women with a High-Risk Pregnancy

A high-risk pregnancy refers to a pregnancy in which the mother or infant has a higher risk of health complications. This may include disorders such as preeclampsia, gestational diabetes, multiple gestations, and premature labor. Women with a high-risk pregnancy may need to take additional measures when it comes to activity and diet. Here are some considerations:

1. **Talk with a healthcare practitioner:** Women with a high-risk pregnancy should work closely with a healthcare professional to build a strategy for managing their pregnancy. This may entail monitoring weight growth, maintaining a certain diet, and exercising consistently. A healthcare practitioner may give recommendations on healthy exercise and diet depending on the woman's unique circumstances.

2. **Diet:** A nutritious, well-balanced diet is vital for women with high-risk pregnancies. Women should attempt to consume a range of meals from all food categories to ensure they are receiving the nutrients they need for a healthy pregnancy. Depending on the woman's health, a

qualified dietitian may be contacted to establish a food plan that matches their requirements.

3. **Exercise:** Exercise may assist improve general health throughout pregnancy, but women with a high-risk pregnancy may need to adapt their exercise program as their pregnancy continues. Depending on the woman's health, exercise may need to be reduced or avoided completely. Women with a high-risk pregnancy should contact their healthcare physician before commencing an exercise regimen.

4. **Monitoring weight increase:** Women with a high-risk pregnancy may need to monitor their weight growth more carefully than women with a low-risk pregnancy. Women should strive to gain weight at a regular rate during their pregnancy, although the quantity of weight increase will vary based on their specific circumstances. Healthcare practitioners may assist select an acceptable weight gain target.

5. **Rest:** Women with a high-risk pregnancy may require more rest than those with a low-risk pregnancy. It is crucial to listen to the body and relax when required to avoid difficulties during pregnancy.

6. **Medications:** Women with a high-risk pregnancy may need to take drugs to control their condition. Certain drugs

might decrease appetite; therefore, it is vital to consult with a healthcare professional and certified dietitian to ensure enough nutrition is maintained.

7. **Monitoring blood sugar:** Women with gestational diabetes or other diseases that influence blood sugar may need to check their blood sugar levels frequently and follow a particular diet to manage their condition.

In summary, women with a high-risk pregnancy may need to take additional measures when it comes to activity and diet. By working together with a healthcare professional and qualified dietitian, clients may build a plan that matches their particular requirements and guarantees a safe pregnancy and birth.

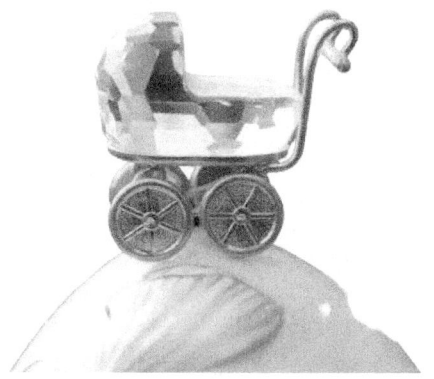

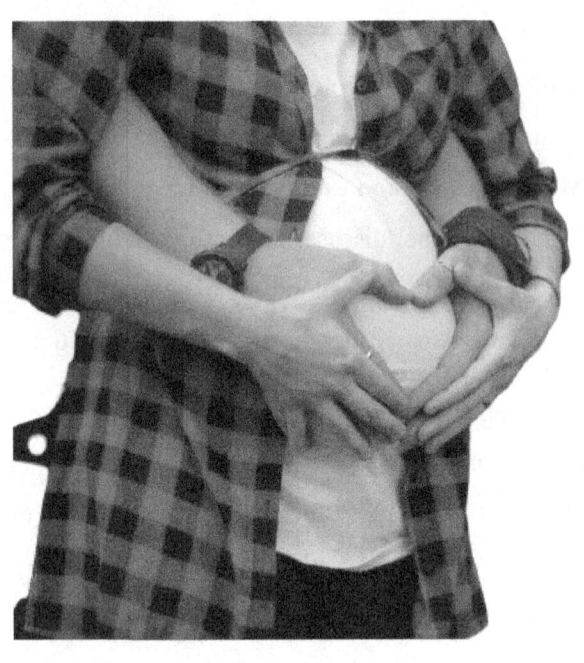

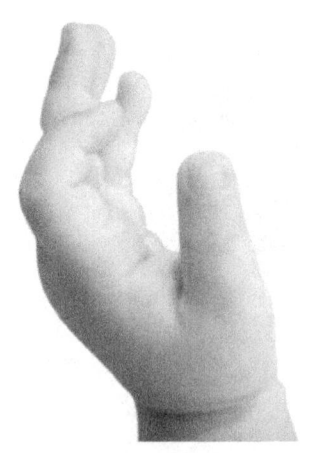

CHAPTER SIX

Postpartum Fitness and Nutrition

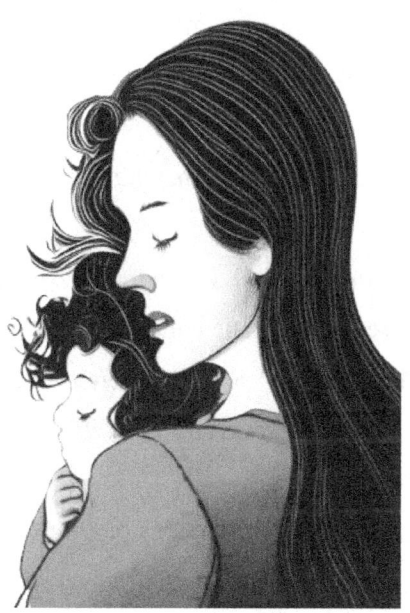

Postpartum exercise and nutrition are vital to the rehabilitation of the body after delivery. A good diet and exercise may help new moms restore their strength, energy, and general health. In this section, we will explore the advantages of postpartum fitness and nutrition, as well as advice for safely introducing exercise and good eating habits into your routine.

Advantages of Postpartum Fitness and Nutrition

The postpartum period may be physically and emotionally hard for new moms. But, taking care of your body with exercise and an adequate diet may have various advantages, including:

1. **Faster recovery:** Exercise and diet may assist speed up the recovery process after delivery, as it helps to boost blood flow and oxygen supply to the mending tissues.

2. **Improved energy levels:** Postpartum exercise may assist to raise energy levels, making it simpler to take care of a baby.

3. **Better mood:** Exercise and good eating habits may help to decrease stress and enhance overall mood.

4. **Improved sleep:** Regular exercise and a good diet may also help to improve sleep quality, which is vital for new moms.

5. **Weight management:** Postpartum exercise and a good diet may help new moms reduce weight accumulated during pregnancy and maintain a healthy weight.

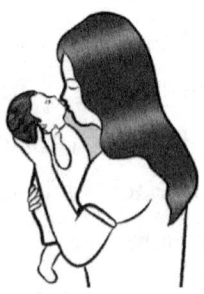

Suggestions for Postpartum Exercise

It is vital to wait until your doctor gives you the green light before commencing any fitness plan after delivery. Generally, this is approximately six weeks postpartum. But every woman's recovery is different, so be sure to consult with your doctor before beginning any exercise regimen.

Here are some guidelines for properly adding fitness into your postpartum routine:

1. **Start slow:** Begin with mild workouts such as walking or easy stretching. Gradually increase the intensity and length of your exercises.

2. **Concentrate on your core:** Pregnancy may weaken your core muscles, so it is crucial to add activities that target these muscles, such as pelvic tilts and Kegels.

3. **Exercise excellent posture:** Bad posture may contribute to back pain and other discomforts, so are sure to practice good posture while exercising and throughout the day.

4. **Listen to your body:** Take attention to how you feel during and after exercise. If you feel any pain or discomfort, stop and speak to your doctor.

5. **Keep hydrated:** Drink lots of water before, during, and after exercise to remain hydrated.

Suggestions for Postpartum Nutrition

A good diet is also vital for postpartum healing. Here are some guidelines for a good diet after childbirth:

1. **Have a balanced diet:** Be sure to consume a range of nutrient-rich foods, including fruits, vegetables, whole grains, lean meats, and healthy fats.

2. **Keep hydrated:** Drink lots of water and other hydrating drinks throughout the day.

3. **Avoid restrictive diets:** Avoid fad diets or tight eating regimens, since they may be damaging to your health and impair milk production.

4. **Eat enough calories:** Breastfeeding moms need an extra 500 calories per day to sustain milk production and support their energy demands.

5. **Plan:** Meal planning may help you keep on track with good eating habits, particularly during the hectic postpartum time.

Postpartum exercise and nutrition are vital for new moms' general health and well-being. By combining regular exercise and a healthy, balanced diet into your routine, you may speed up your recuperation, enhance your energy levels, and control your weight.

Remember to speak with your doctor before beginning any fitness program and make sure to listen to your body throughout exercises. With patience and effort, you may successfully navigate the postpartum period and have a healthy, happy life with your new baby.

Exercise Guidelines and Considerations After Pregnancy

So, after pregnancy, your body needs time to recuperate from the physical changes and demands of delivery. It's crucial to allow yourself to relax and recuperate before entering into any intense fitness plan. Your doctor will typically suggest waiting at least 6 weeks before beginning exercise, however, this might vary based on specific circumstances.

After you have been approved to exercise, it's vital to start cautiously and gradually build intensity and length over time. Some suggested workouts for postpartum women include:

1. **Walking:** Walking is a low-impact exercise that can be done practically any place and is a fantastic way to ease back into physical activity after delivery.
2. **Pelvic floor exercises:** These exercises serve to strengthen the muscles that support the bladder, uterus,

and rectum. These may be done anywhere and at any time, making them a simple addition to your regular regimen.

3. **Yoga:** Yoga may assist to develop flexibility and strength, while also lowering tension and fostering relaxation. Postpartum yoga sessions generally concentrate on poses that are safe for new moms and their newborns.

4. **Strength training:** Strength training may assist to tone and strengthen your muscles, which can be particularly advantageous after pregnancy and delivery.

5. **Swimming:** Swimming is a low-impact activity that may be particularly good for ladies healing after a cesarean section.

It's crucial to listen to your body and cease any workout that produces pain or discomfort. If you develop any unexpected symptoms such as bleeding, dizziness, or shortness of breath, stop exercising and see your doctor.

In addition to exercise, diet is also vital for postpartum recovery. It's crucial to consume a balanced diet that contains lots of fruits, vegetables, whole grains, lean meats, and healthy fats. Breastfeeding women should strive to eat an additional 500 calories each day to promote milk production.

It's also crucial to remain hydrated by drinking lots of water and other drinks. Avoid sugary beverages and restrict your caffeine consumption, since too much caffeine might interfere with your sleep and hydration levels.

Exercise and diet are crucial components of postpartum rehabilitation. By beginning gently and progressively increasing intensity, you may safely resume physical exercise after delivery. Consuming a balanced diet and being hydrated will also assist to promote your body's recovery and ensuring that you have the energy and nutrition you need to care for yourself and your new baby.

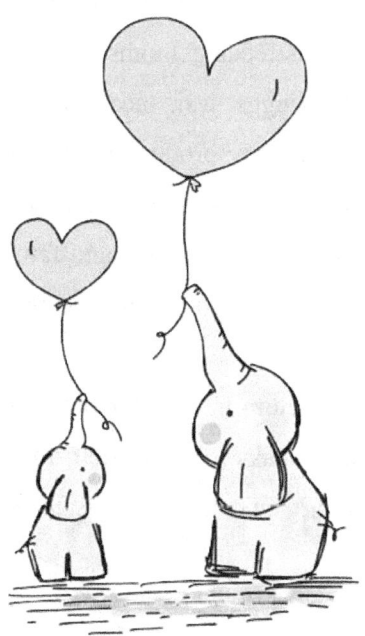

Nutrition Recommendations for Breastfeeding Moms

A good diet is vital for nursing women since it encourages the production of breast milk and delivers nutrients to the infant. Breastfeeding moms need an extra 450 to 500 calories per day to guarantee they have enough energy to make milk and nurture their babies.

These are some dietary guidelines for nursing moms:

1. **Hydrate:** Drinking adequate water is vital for nursing women. It is essential to drink at least 8-10 glasses of water every day to keep hydrated.

2. **Protein:** Breastfeeding moms should take protein-rich foods such as eggs, lean meats, fish, lentils, and dairy products to boost the production of breast milk.

3. **Healthy fats:** Breastfeeding moms should eat healthy fats such as avocado, nuts, seeds, and fatty fish to boost the baby's brain development and the production of breast milk.

4. **Calcium:** Calcium is vital for bone health, and nursing moms should take calcium-rich foods such as milk, cheese, yogurt, and leafy greens to achieve their daily needs.

5. **Iron:** Nursing moms need more iron to restore the iron lost after delivery and to assist the baby's development. Iron-rich foods such as lean meats, beans, nuts, and leafy greens should be incorporated into the diet.

6. **Fruits and veggies:** Breastfeeding women should eat a range of fruits and vegetables to give the required vitamins and minerals for both themselves and their infant.

7. **Avoid specific meals:** Certain foods may transfer into breast milk and trigger bad effects in newborns, including coffee, spicy foods, and alcohol. It is suggested to restrict or avoid certain meals during nursing.

In addition to a nutritious diet, nursing women should also take care of themselves by obtaining adequate rest and exercise. Mild to moderate exercise may help enhance mood and energy levels and promote milk production.

It is vital to contact a healthcare physician or a trained dietitian for individualized dietary advice for nursing women.

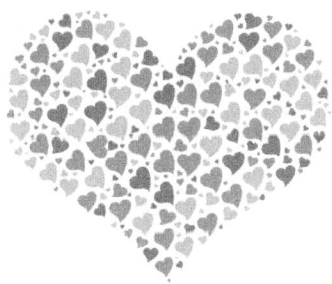

Sample Meal Plans for Postpartum Recovery

After giving delivery, it is crucial to continue eating a well-balanced diet to aid postpartum healing and nursing. Here are some example meal plans to aid you in planning your postpartum diet:

DAY 1:

Breakfast:

- Oatmeal with sliced banana, chopped almonds, and a drizzle of honey, served with a cup of green tea.

Snack: Apple slices with almond butter.

Lunch:

- Grilled chicken salad with mixed greens, cherry tomatoes, avocado, and balsamic vinaigrette dressing.

Snack: Greek yogurt with sliced strawberries and a sprinkling of granola.

Dinner:

- Grilled salmon with roasted veggies (zucchini, carrots, and bell peppers) and quinoa.

DAY 2:

Breakfast:

- Whole wheat bread with scrambled eggs and sautéed spinach, accompanied by a cup of coffee.

Snack: Tiny carrots with hummus.

Lunch:

- Lentil soup with a side of whole-grain crackers and mixed fruit salad.

Snack: Cottage cheese with sliced peaches and a dab of honey.

Dinner:

- Roasted chicken breast with roasted sweet potato wedges and a side of green beans.

DAY 3:

Breakfast:

- Whole-grain waffle with almond butter and sliced banana, accompanied by a cup of herbal tea.

Snack: Edamame beans.

Lunch:

- Tuna salad sandwich on whole-grain bread with a side of mixed greens and cherry tomatoes.

Snack: Baked sweet potato with a dollop of Greek yogurt and a sprinkling of cinnamon.

Dinner:

- Turkey chili with mixed vegetables and a side of brown rice.

DAY 4:

Breakfast:

- Greek yogurt with mixed berries and a sprinkling of chia seeds, served with a cup of green tea.

Snack: Roasted pumpkin seeds.

Lunch:

- Grilled chicken wrap with mixed greens, avocado, and hummus, served with a side of fruit salad.

Snack: Banana with almond butter and a dab of honey.

Dinner:

- Grilled shrimp with mixed veggies (broccoli, carrots, and snow peas) with a side of quinoa.

DAY 5:

Breakfast:

- Scrambled eggs with whole-grain bread and a side of fruit salad, served with a cup of coffee.

Snack: Celery sticks with peanut butter.

Lunch:

- Vegetarian burger with a side of roasted sweet potato wedges and mixed greens salad.

Snack: Chopped vegetables (cucumber, carrot, and bell pepper) with hummus.

Dinner:

- Baked salmon with roasted asparagus and a dish of brown rice.

Note: These are simply samples of sample meal plans, and it's crucial to personalize them depending on your specific tastes, dietary requirements, and food intolerances. It's also vital to talk with your healthcare physician before making any big adjustments to your postpartum diet.

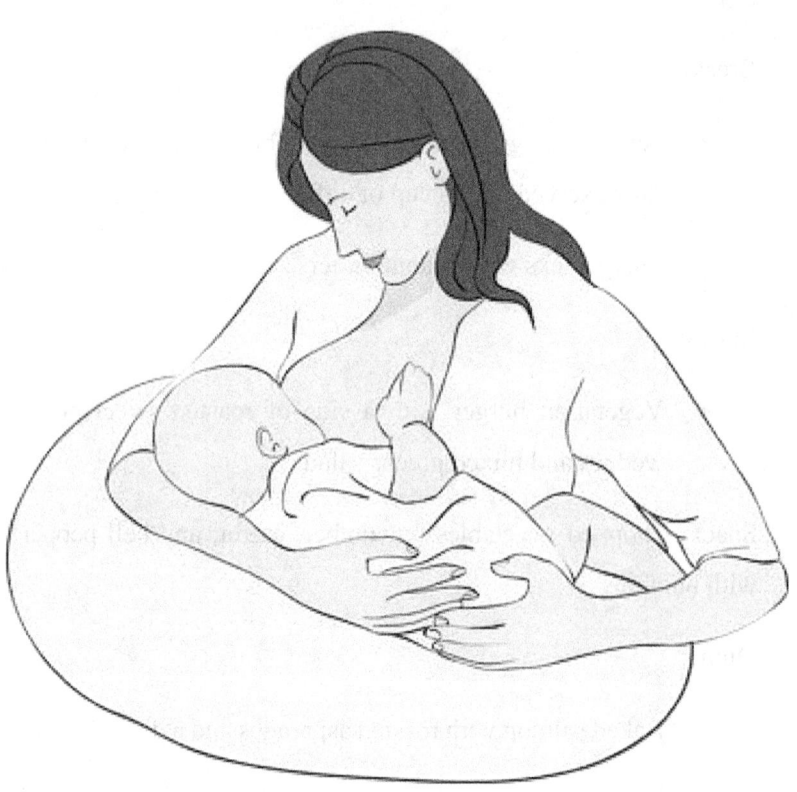

CONCLUSION

Congrats on finishing "Fit for Two: A Comprehensive Workout and Food Plan Guide for Expectant Moms"! By reading this book, you have made a vital step towards having a successful pregnancy and postpartum recovery. Remember that being active and eating a balanced diet are vital components of a healthy pregnancy and may have great benefits for both you and your baby.

Throughout this book, we have covered the benefits of exercise and proper nutrition during pregnancy, the changes in the body during pregnancy, recommended exercise guidelines, nutrition requirements during pregnancy, macronutrients and micronutrients for a healthy pregnancy, exercise during pregnancy, meal planning for a healthy pregnancy, building a balanced pregnancy meal plan, managing pregnancy cravings and aversions, special considerations during pregnancy, and postpartum fitness and nutrition.

It is vital to bear in mind that every pregnancy is unique and individual demands may differ. Be cautious to contact your healthcare practitioner before beginning any fitness program or making changes to your diet. They may give you unique advice depending on your medical history and personal requirements.

We hope that this book has given you helpful knowledge and resources to help you have a good pregnancy and postpartum recovery. Remember to listen to your body and make alterations as required. With determination and perseverance, you should attain a healthy and fit pregnancy!

Maintaining a Healthy Lifestyle After Pregnancy

After giving birth, it is crucial to continue to focus on your health and welfare. Here are some ideas for keeping a healthy lifestyle after pregnancy:

1. **Ease back into exercise:** Your body has gone through a lot of changes and it is important to ease back into exercise to avoid injury. Start with low-impact workouts and progressively increase intensity and duration over time. Be mindful to listen to your body and take pauses as required.

2. **Keep hydrated:** Consuming adequate water is vital for your general health and may assist with milk production if you are nursing. Carry a water bottle with you throughout the day and strive to drink at least 8-10 glasses of water every day.

3. **Get enough sleep:** Lack of sleep can impact your physical and mental health, so it is important to prioritize sleep. Try to establish a sleep routine and nap when you can to make up for any lost sleep.

4. **Continue to eat a balanced diet:** Your body needs nourishment to recover from childbirth and support breastfeeding if applicable. Continue to eat a balanced diet with a variety of fruits, vegetables, whole grains, and lean proteins.

5. **Seek support:** Taking care of a newborn can be overwhelming, so it is important to seek support from family, friends, or a healthcare provider if needed. Attending a support group or interacting with other new parents may also be beneficial.

Remember that taking care of yourself is important not just for your health, but for the health of your baby as well. By continuing to prioritize exercise, nutrition, and self-care, you can maintain a healthy lifestyle after pregnancy.

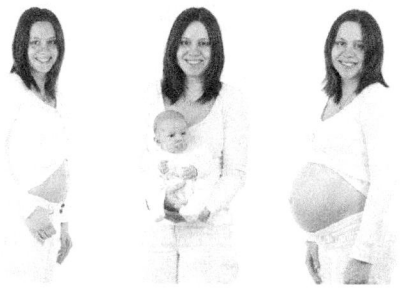

Final Thoughts and Encouragement

Remember, taking care of yourself at this time is not only vital for your health but also for the health of your kid. By following the fitness and diet instructions in this book, you will be setting yourself up for success and giving your kid the greatest possible start in life.

Lastly, I want to urge you to continue living a healthy lifestyle following pregnancy. By making exercise and good eating a priority in your life, you will not only be establishing a wonderful example for your children but also boosting your lifespan and quality of life.

Thank you for reading "Fit for Two: A Comprehensive Workout and Food Plan Guide for Expectant Moms." I wish you all the best on your pregnancy and parenthood journey.

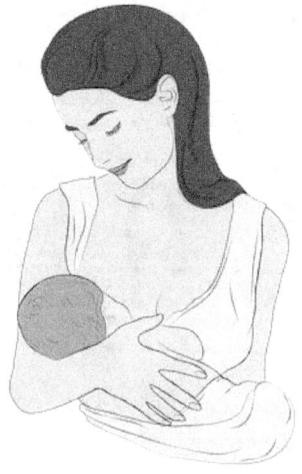

Mood Tracker

	J	F	M	A	M	J	J	A	S	O	N	D
1												
2												
3												
4												
5												
6												
7												
8												
9												
10												
11												
12												
13												
14												
15												
16												
17												
18												
19												
20												
21												
22												
23												
24												
25												
26												
27												
28												
29												
30												
31												

Assign color and mood to a specific square
and color the squares according to
your mood

Mood Tracker

	J	F	M	A	M	J	J	A	S	O	N	D
1												
2												
3												
4												
5												
6												
7												
8												
9												
10												
11												
12												
13												
14												
15												
16												
17												
18												
19												
20												
21												
22												
23												
24												
25												
26												
27												
28												
29												
30												
31												

Assign color and mood to a specific square
and color the squares according to
your mood

WORKOUT LOG

NAME:_____

GOALS:_____

DATE:

STATS:

WEIGHT:

EXERCISE:	SETS	REPS	WEIGHT	REST	SETS	REPS	WEIGHT	REST	SETS	REPS	WEIGHT	REST	SETS	REPS	WEIGHT	REST

CARDIO:	TIME	DIST.	INT.	PACE	TIME	DIST.	INT.	PACE	TIME	DIST.	INT.	PACE	TIME	DIST.	INT.	PACE

WORKOUT LOG

NAME:_____

GOALS:_____

DATE:

STATS:

WEIGHT:

EXERCISE:	SETS	REPS	WEIGHT	REST	SETS	REPS	WEIGHT	REST	SETS	REPS	WEIGHT	REST	SETS	REPS	WEIGHT	REST

CARDIO:	TIME	DIST.	INT.	PACE	TIME	DIST.	INT.	PACE	TIME	DIST.	INT.	PACE	TIME	DIST.	INT.	PACE

SIMPLE WEIGHT TRACKER

DATE	TIME	WEIGHT	NOTES / COMMENTS

SIMPLE WEIGHT TRACKER

DATE	TIME	WEIGHT	NOTES / COMMENTS

Made in the USA
Middletown, DE
08 October 2025

18971714R00076